THE NEW
CONTROLLED CHEATING
WEIGHT-LOSS AND FITNESS PROGRAM

THE NEW
CONTROLLED
CHEATING

WEIGHT-LOSS AND
FITNESS PROGRAM

or

How I Lost 175 Pounds and Kept It Off for 32 Years.

BY LARRY **FATS** GOLDBERG

Andrews and McMeel

A Universal Press Syndicate Company

Kansas City

Designed by Barrie Maguire

Library of Congress Cataloging-in-Publication Data

Goldberg, Larry, 1934–
    The new controlled chEATing weight-loss and fitness program, or,
How I lost 175 pounds and kept it off for 32 years /
by Larry FATS Goldberg.
    p. cm.
    ISBN 0-8362-2419-1 (ppb) : $9.95
    1. Reducing. 2. Reducing diets. I. Title. II. Title: How I
lost 175 pounds and kept it off for 32 years.
    RM222.2.G595   1991
    613.2'5—dc20   91-30639
                                                            CIP

Attention: Schools and Businesses

Andrews and McMeel books are available at quantity discounts with bulk purchase for educational, business, or sales promotional use. For information, please write to: Special Sales Department, Andrews and McMeel, 4900 Main Street, Kansas City, Missouri 64112.

CONTENTS

ACKNOWLEDGMENTS

Rochelle Larkin, friend and writer, who said,
"Goldberg, write this book!"

Donna Martin, friend and editor, who said,
"Goldberg, do some work!"

Kathryn Kreider, friend and computer tamer, who said,
"Goldberg, write it, I'll type it!"

DEDICATION

For my folks

Sara and Art Goldberg, my sister Joc,
whose money I snitched as a kid so I could eat more and ...

Goldberg's Market
"Fancy Groceries and Meats, Free Delivery (me), Call WA 0030"
3843 Agnes, Kansas City, Missouri

YOU'D
BETTER
READ
THIS

I'm taking one whole page—and pages cost much money—to tell you something. No, more than tell you—beseech you, command you. And you'd better damn well do what I tell you!

Before you do anything in this book:

GO TO YOUR DOCTOR
AND DISCUSS CONTROLLED CHEATING
WITH HIM OR HER!

I'm going to repeat this throughout the book until you're sick of it, but it's your health I'm worried about.

P.S. I do not work for the American Medical Association.

FOREWORD

I remember the day I first met Larry Goldberg in my office. During the interview, as he revealed to me his history of tremendous weight loss, I was very impressed that he had been able to keep it off. This was surprising in light of the fact that he "loves to eat." Before too long I found out I was talking to "Fats" Goldberg, the author of *Controlled Cheating*. I had read the first edition of his book several years earlier and it made a very positive impression on me. I had recommended his book and the philosophy of a "cheater's diet" to many of my patients. I always thought it was the most sensible approach to dieting.

In my years of practice I have prescribed weight loss to countless numbers of patients. The most common medical problems that respond to weight loss are hypertension, elevated cholesterol, and diabetes mellitus. Obviously, many people with coronary artery disease, osteoarthritis, and musculo-skeletal symptoms also would benefit from weight reduction. Relatively few actually lose enough weight to have a significant impact on their health, and most of those that do eventually gain the weight back. The secret to successful dieting is not in any special food preparation, liquid protein mixture, or quick weight loss gimmicks. What is needed is a change in lifestyle!

Pharmaceutical companies have known for a long time that their most popular medications are the ones accepted by patients willingly. More importantly, the patients must be committed to staying on the medication for years. Virtually all of the leading medications are now made in "once a day" formulations. This has greatly enhanced compliance. Compliance is the key to a successful weight loss program as well.

Larry Goldberg has developed a diet program that is readily accepted and easily adhered to. He supplies the reader with the facts needed along with a sense of humor. "Fats" Goldberg lost 175 pounds and has kept it off. He is an enthusiastic and vigorous individual. His diet program is healthy and medically sound, and he has a unique approach to weight loss.

Alexander C. Davis, M.D.
Internal Medicine
Kansas City, Missouri

CONTROLLED CHEATING

OR

HOW I LOST 175 POUNDS
AND KEPT IT OFF
FOR THIRTY-TWO YEARS

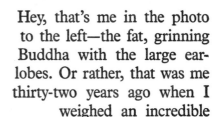

Hey, that's me in the photo to the left—the fat, grinning Buddha with the large earlobes. Or rather, that was me thirty-two years ago when I weighed an incredible 325 pounds in my hometown of Kansas City. The slim matinee idol on p. 212 is me, too—last month when I slipped in at 160 pounds. I've lost a whole Goldberg. But my pal's ready to come back to life any time I slide back to my old gorging habits.

I LOVE TO EAT. Even the word "food" conjures up dreams of grease, dough, and sugar.

When I was twenty-two and had just graduated from college, I had a complete physical, the first one of my life. After some horrible tests, the doctor took me into his office, shut the door, and gravely announced that I had diabetes (of the latent variety). My three double chins started to tremble; I was terrified. But, he said, I could cure my diabetes through diet. I regained my composure, straightened my tummy, and then walked out the door, got in my car, and drove to Winstead's Drive-In. I ate three double cheeseburgers with grilled onions, two fresh-lime Cokes, and a Frosty Malt. When I was heavy and got hungry, the angel of death could be sitting on my shoulder and I wouldn't miss a bite.

Oh boy. Unfortunately for most fatties, it's the old story of laughing through the tears. And the world doesn't make it any easier. First of all, we have to eat every day to live. Even worse, when I walk down any street, I see and smell pizzerias, delicatessens, Baskin-Robbinses, and mall food courts. Food surrounds us. Food is cheap. And you don't have to be twenty-one.

I was born fifty-seven years ago, to Sara and Art Goldberg of Kansas City, Missouri. I weighed seven pounds, fourteen ounces. Sara, who weighed 140 pounds, was the Jelly Bean Queen of Kansas City. She used to hang around Woolworth's candy counter eating candy orange slices. Art weighed 150 pounds, never got hungry, and owned a small food emporium called (big surprise) "Goldberg's Market—Fancy Groceries and Meats," with free delivery (I was the free delivery). Jocelyn, my sister, is five years older than me . . . and skinny. Lucky Joc.

Ma says I was a "chunky" baby, and that I was eating everything in sight while I was still gurgling in her arms. My earliest recorded weight was in the third grade, 105 pounds. By eighth grade, I weighed a cool 240 pounds. When Ma would cook she'd make six pork chops; one for each of them and three for me. I was so "chunky" I couldn't sit in a normal desk. Mrs. Burns, my teacher, had me sit in a straight chair on the side of the room.

My ace pediatrician once hauled me up on the table when I was a little fat kid and said, "Do you want to die in ten years?"

This is when the diets started. Every doctor would gaze at my stomach and give me a mimeographed sheet with sample diets. I'd drag the diet home, diet through breakfast, and blow the whole mess at lunch.

My parents couldn't stop me from eating—no one could. They'd have had to keep an eye on me twenty-four hours a day. If I couldn't eat at home or in the grocery store, I'd eat at a neighbor's, at a friend's house, or with strangers.

Popping prescribed diet pills came during my freshman year of high school. I ran the whole diet pill string, from the worthless ones through the powerful Dexedrine spansules that made me giggle a lot. None worked for long. The minute I'd stop taking the pills, I'd start eating all over again. The only real difference in my life was that by now I was terrified all the time, a perpetual hypochondriac.

High school was a lot of laughs. I bought a '37 Oldsmobile that started leaning toward the left. Anyone who sat next to me automatically slid down to my side on the nylon seat cover. That could have been exciting, except I had only two dates in high school.

Actually, there was one other date in high school—the Sunday school confirmation dance. Everyone in the class had dates except me and Minnie Plotz. Poor Minnie was almost as fat as I was, so the Sunday school teacher arranged the fix-up. We danced once. That was the first time I'd ever held a girl in my arms—also the first time I'd ever danced. But we were so big our extended arms could barely touch each other's sides.

My official weight when I graduated from high school and got my draft card was 265 pounds. Kansas City Junior College was next.

During my first year I sold ladies' shoes at a local Baker's Shoe Store and earned my nickname, "Three Cases Goldberg." Selling a "case" in shoe peddling meant selling a hundred dollars' worth of shoes. For me, though, the name applied not to my sales, but to my size—three-hundred-pound Goldberg.

In college, guys are supposed to become clothes-conscious, but I did all my fancy dressing at Sears or the local army-navy store. They were the only places that could fit me. My costume never varied. First I wore Sears Roebuck's "Armored Crotch" boxer shorts. They were reinforced between the legs because you know how fat boys chafe. Then I wore eighteen-inch-neck white or blue oxford-cloth button-down shirts. I was a three-hundred-pound sex bomb in saddle shoes.

Off to the University of Missouri to journalism school, and I pledged Zeta Beta Tau fraternity. There I went formal and started wearing fifty-inch-waist khakis. I now weighed 305 pounds and had managed to kiss one girl, once.

I always tried to take a shower alone in the fraternity house because I was embarrassed by my size. One day I happened to glance at my naked body after taking a shower. I noticed a string of little red scratches circling my tummy. Although I tried never to look at myself completely undressed, now that I had done so, panic set in. I ran to the doctor, who told me those red lines were stretch marks. That is, the skin couldn't hold the fat. He reassured me that they were harmless and that pregnant women get them all the time. But, I moaned, I wasn't a pregnant woman. After that, when anyone saw me naked, I told them I fought tigers in the circus during the summer. I was thoroughly depressed until I could get to a pint of butterscotch swirl ice cream.

Once during my first year, after I had eaten three complete lunches in one hour, I thought I had finally done it: I was going to explode and die from overeating. Struggling over to the infirmary, I bared my soul to the doctor. I begged him for a diet. Being more accustomed to mononucleosis than obesity, he pushed his finger in my stomach, shook his head, told me to cool it on the groceries, and gave me a can of foot powder.

The worst night I ever spent during my fat years was in the fraternity house. I started salivating around eight-thirty at night, waiting for the sandwich man who came around at ten o'clock. But that night he didn't show. By eleven-thirty I was in a state of hungry panic. Everything in Columbia, Missouri, was closed except for the doughnut shop downtown, and to top it all off, it was snowing. I ran from room to room, sweating and screaming for someone to take me to eat. At last, Dave Goodman, God bless

him, took pity on my crazed condition and drove me to the Broadway Donut Shop for a dozen hot glazed doughnuts and a quart of
chocolate milk. I stopped twitching.

The first year after I graduated from college in journalism, I
had four jobs. I counted Japanese thong sandals in bins, sold
radio time for a rock station in Kansas City, went back to Columbia as a radio announcer (calling myself Fats Goldberg, the Sheik
of Columbia), and was a television announcer, off camera, of
course. Finally I wound up in Chicago working for the *Chicago
Tribune*, and it was there that I made a decision. I was really tired
of being fat. I was uncomfortable, the morning heartburn really
hurt, and being fat was rapidly becoming no fun.

On Monday, May 1, 1959, I awoke and rubbed my food-
swollen eyes and said to myself, "Today's the day I'm going to
start my diet." I'd said these words to myself almost every morning since the day I was born.

The last time I'd weighed myself was three or four years
before when I'd found a freight and cattle scale. (Household scales,
at least the ones I've seen, go only to three hundred pounds.) I'd
hopped on the freight scale, and when the needle started careen-
ing over three hundred and wasn't slowing down, I leapt off. It
had hit 325, but I really didn't know how much I weighed. I could
have been close to four "cases."

On the first day of the rest of my life, I rolled out of bed and
took one of those Dexedrine spansule diet pills. After a breakfast
of two scrambled eggs, an English muffin, and two cups of coffee,
I decided there'd be no more diet pills. Either I was going to do
this cold turkey, just me and my stomach, or I'd just keep eating
until my navel popped out and I'd die, having lived a short, fat
life.

For lunch, I had to meet a used car dealer to whom I was
trying to sell ad space in the *Chicago Tribune*, and he wanted to go
to a smorgasbord. What a way to start a diet! But I ate only a
couple of pieces of roast beef and a few green beans. And for
dinner I held myself to steak and cottage cheese.

The first three letters of diet are *d-i-e*. On the second day of
dieting, I believed death would have been easier. I didn't think I

could take dieting any longer. With no exaggeration, my whole body from my hair to my corns craved and demanded food. Still, I gritted my underused teeth and somehow stuck it out.

At 325 pounds, 190 was my goal, but it seemed to be a life-time away. It had taken me twenty-five years to put that weight on, and I wanted to take it off in three days. The second week I lost seventeen pounds. I didn't care if it was water or cheesecake, I was losing weight. This made me feel great. I was accomplishing something. I could feel it, and I could see it when I got on the scale.

When I made that decision to diet, I had to make a total commitment to a new life-style. If I was going to lose weight, I had to stop eating. So when the hunger pains were making my stomach do Rock Around the Clock, I would think about Cater-pillar tractors, joint sessions of Congress, Marilyn Monroe—any-thing except food.

I read that the healthy way to eat was to breakfast like a king, lunch like a prince, and dine like a pauper. I used that system for years and it works, though I've now developed Goldberg's varia-tions. I would get up in the morning, drink a glass of skim milk to get me rolling, then follow it with two eggs, toast, and coffee. Lunch was a sandwich and a glass of milk. I always took the top piece of bread off and folded the two halves together. That way I saved the calories in a slice of bread. Dinner was red meat of some kind, or chicken or turkey, with cottage cheese or tomato. No one knew of cholesterol in those days. Cholesterol was something you cleaned the kitchen with. You didn't eat fiber, you made clothes out of it. High protein diets were the style.

Putting variety in my diet was hard. I used to find a food that would let me lose weight and I'd eat so much of it, I'd get to the point where I couldn't stand to look at it anymore. Take fresh pineapple. It was juicy, cold, and sweet, and it filled me up. But I ate so much, leaves started growing out of my head. I also ate tons of cottage cheese and my skin started to curdle. Boredom is a dangerous feeling when you're dieting.

Crawling up that slippery road of dieting, my poor vacant tummy got weary of the struggle. And shoot—this was only after the first three weeks. Here I go again; the old diet elevator, the Overweight Otis, the Wagonload Westinghouse, up and down the scale; lose ten, put back fifteen.

After a fast start, I looked at the stormy horizon and saw that nothing good to eat was in the forecast. I choked back a tear. I knew I had to try a different road.

One day while walking down Michigan Avenue, it hit me like ton of warm glazed doughnuts. I was going to pick one glorious day out of every week and eat anything in the world I wanted. Finally, there was a light at the end of the tunnel, a diet tunnel that was only six days long. Even old weak Fatberg could stay on a mean, dumb diet for six days when there was manna and everything else from heaven on the seventh. This was it—skyrockets going off, fireworks, bands playing—Controlled Cheating was born in a flash.

The first Cheating Day was a Sunday and brought caloric joy to my deprived body. I had pecan pancakes with lots of butter and syrup, pepperoni pizza, hot popcorn, two Pepsis, and a bagel with cream cheese.

Ah, but there was a cigar butt in the banana cream pie. Could I go back on the diet after that one happy Cheating Day?

The next morning I hopped on the scale. Help me God, four pounds gained. My eyes glazed over like doughnuts. With panic and pain, I realized this was the supreme test. I set my quivering jaw and started back into the diet mine shaft. After all, it was only six stinky diet days back to heavenly Sunday.

Looking back over all those dumb diets I could never stay on, I realized that a person can't look down that long road of life and never see another hot fudge sundae. Controlled Cheating was the answer. Strict balanced dieting with nutritious foods for six days, with one day off for gluttonous behavior.

Thirty-two skinny years have convinced me that Controlled Cheating is a weight-loss-and-maintenance plan that can allow any man, woman, or child to lose however much or little he or she wants, and to *maintain that ideal weight*.

My overall goal was to lose 130 of my 325-plus pounds, but, being weak and not knowing how long I could last without a food reward, I set intermediate goals. The first goal was to weigh 265 pounds when I went on vacation to Kansas City after three months of dieting. When I walked in the back door of my house, Ma was peeling potatoes. She looked up and said, "Yes?" For a second, she hadn't even recognized her bouncing baby boy. I was thrilled.

Everywhere, in Chicago and Kansas City, people would notice the difference immediately. My size fifty-two-long suits were getting very baggy. I woke up without heartburn. Everyone was tremendously encouraging, and when they got me alone would ask how I did it. The management at the *Chicago Tribune* became more interested in my career. I was taken off probation on the company's major medical policy. I developed a new self-confidence and outlook on everything, including my social life.

Demon temptations were always around: pungent-smelling fast-food joints, or dinner in a restaurant or someone's house. But I learned how to cope by saying no, unless it was Sunday.

Pain was my constant companion—the physical pain of being hungry and the psychological pain of deprivation. I had to change my life-style to one that wasn't centered around food.

I did it. In one year I lost 130 pounds.

When I weighed 190 pounds, I went into the pizza business in New York City.

I figured that if I couldn't eat it, at least I could become a pizza voyeur, selling and smelling the best and one of the most nutritious foods in the world. A son-of-a-gun-a mozzarella miracle happened. *New York* magazine had a pizza contest, and Goldberg's Pizzeria was voted the best in the Big Apple.

There I was, at the age of thirty-four, crouched in front of two 650-degree ovens schlepping pizzas. The night shift at the steel mill open hearth in Gary, Indiana, was easier. My Health-O-Meter scale started to go down again. Terrific. Now twenty-three years later, I'm down to a constant 160 and lean as a cougar.

It wasn't only sweating that peeled off the last thirty pounds. I became an expert in losing weight, especially on my own personal system. Diet and nutrition books are like fried chicken to me. I can't get enough. But after thirty-two years, the more I read, see, and talk, the more I'm convinced that there is no fast, easy, and painless way to lose weight permanently. Dieting is a job, but as with any job, I discovered I can have days off. That's the beauty of Controlled Cheating and why it works.

The usual history of the dieter is like that of a convict. After getting out of the prison of their fat, they regress and go back behind bars. What I want you to do is melt those nasty fat bars down *permanently*. That's what we're going to do right here.

Controlled Cheating works. But it demands discipline.

Once you pick your Controlled Cheating Day, that day cannot be changed.

I don't care if Christmas falls on a Saturday and your Cheating Day is Sunday, or you are invited to dinner at Julia Child's or you're going home to Mom's apple pie and warm corn bread with sweet butter, or that dynamite woman you've been panting to take out just said yes to dinner—you MUST stick to your plan.

We all have 14 million reasons to go back to stuffing our mouths. There will always be excuses your tummy will broadcast to your brain to be filled up. You cannot change your Cheating Day for every hot excuse that comes along. Before you can say, "Big Mac," you'll be back gorging every day. Buck up, set your jaw, and dream of your coming Diet Oasis.

Cheating once a week, it's easy to stay with this plan for the rest of your life and *never gain weight again.*

The diet-day menu can vary as to time and foods eaten, but I always eat a balanced diet. I eat little meals all through the day. This way I always have something to look forward to. I eat very little red meat on my diet days. And I drink about ten to twelve glasses of water a day. People can always tell when Goldberg dances down the street: they hear the sound of sloshing.

Here are some rules I've set up for myself on my diet days:

1. Exercise.
2. I eliminate all of the fat I can.
3. Eat a high-fiber, low-fat, complex-carbohydrate, balanced diet from all of the food groups.
4. Drink plenty of water.
5. Be flexible. Add a variety of low-calorie foods to the diet.

Boredom in eating the same foods every day is dangerous for a fatty.

6. Eat slowly—I put the fork DOWN after every bite and do not pick the fork up again until after I swallow. Before I lost weight, I ate like a runaway windmill—one whirling, continuous circular motion from the plate to my mouth and back again as fast as I could.

Still, by eleven o'clock, I'm against the wall with hunger. Sometimes it gets so bad that I can't wait to brush my teeth, so I can at least get the taste of toothpaste.

I also dream of food. (I have this recurring dream of bakeries. . . .) Sometimes I wake up feeling sorry for myself. But I have fifty-seven years of a healthy life behind me, and I remind myself that I probably ate more in my first twenty-five years than a normal person would eat in a lifetime. I feel better when I look at it that way.

For years, I saw myself as a trim Burt Lancaster or a rugged Gary Cooper. Right now I'm svelte, but I'll never be rugged. And as for shoulders, I didn't come equipped with any. My exercise consists of riding a stationary bicycle and aerobic dancing. I also do lots of walking—a fast three or four miles a day. This keeps me in pretty good shape, and keeps my podiatrist happy.

There you have it—the way I live and diet. The diet path I've chosen works for me. My fat outlook on life has changed to slim. I am finally a "normal" person, though "normality" was a shock at first.

As a fat man I was safe. That big wall of fat protected me. While other kids were going through the trials of puberty and dating, I escaped by eating my way through adolescence. No wonder I didn't go through puberty until I was thirty-one. No one could get close to me, literally and figuratively. Kidding and teasing were important to keep people away. But now that I'm slim, I don't have to hide behind my fat. I'm more honest about how I feel. And this gives me something I never had—self-confidence. I have become more relaxed and self-assured. Other people look at me with respect, which is a totally new sensation.

After going through the disciplines of dieting, I feel there is nothing I can't handle. In my B.C.C. (Before Controlled Cheating) days, I couldn't call a woman for a date without the phone sliding out of my sweaty hand. Not that I became a swaggering boulevardier or a Robert Redford overnight, but my social life *is* a social life, a full and happy one, not a bunch of excuses and alibis hiding behind a wall of fat.

There are also other big bonuses. I can go into The Gap without the salesman giggling, snorting, and hiding behind the crew-neck sweaters. I can sleep on my stomach without having a stomach ache in the morning. I've stopped gnawing my fingernails. I can wear T-shirts without looking like two St. Bernards in a bag fighting it out. I have a hundred times more energy and require three hours less sleep. I can tie my shoes without crossing my legs. I can sit in a movie theater seat straight and not on my side. People will sit next to me on the bus. I don't sweat as much. Women look at me once in a while on the street. Clothes don't wear out as fast. I can see and feel my bones. I can get in and out of the smallest cars. I even bought a Honda. I have stopped snoring. Sometimes someone says I am too slim and should eat more. I can be the last one on a crowded elevator.

Plus, I recently moved back to Kansas City from New York, so now I can get something really good to eat.

AND if I live even one minute longer because I lost weight, it was all worth it.

WHAT
CONTROLLED
CHEATING
CAN DO FOR YOU

Fats Goldberg's Controlled Cheating

This is the Fats Goldberg Story,
He was the only mountain in Missouri
To curb his overeating
He created Controlled Cheating
Now he's nothing but skin, bones, and glory.

MOST WEIGHT CONTROL SYSTEMS DON'T ALLOW FOR THE POSSIBILITY OF CHEATING. MINE IS BASED ON THE CERTAINTY OF IT.

Controlled Cheating is a different kind of weight loss program. The diet is different. The cheating is different. Plus the whole program is different. Controlled Cheating starts where other diets stop.

We all know people who can eat everything they want and still remain slim. It's not fair, but it's true. The rest of us live a different life. If we eat the foods we love, we gain weight. A little at a time. Say a quarter of a pound a week. Even that adds up to thirteen pounds a year!

So then we try to diet; crash diets, fad diets, powders, shakes, fasting, pills, shots. Whenever we eat less, we lose weight. Then we give in to our cravings and we have a hot fudge sundae or a sack of cookies, and we begin the weight gain all over again. Controlled Cheating offers a true alternative without the tight, restrictive commitments that other weight loss programs require.

Controlled Cheating accepts the fact that you love food, and

13

that you're going to eat the things you love, one way or the other. And that it's okay! Food is not evil. Controlled Cheating actually encourages you to cheat on your diet, but in a controlled way that really makes sense.

You already know how to cheat. You're an expert. You probably know how to diet. I teach you how to put them both together. You will use your Cheating Day to keep yourself on your diet. This all results in a diet program that is actually fun, realistic, and livable. The diet itself is sensible and nutritious with REAL FOOD. Controlled Cheating is inner ecology.

You lose weight slo-o-owly, with a nutritious high-complex-carbohydrate, low-fat, low-sodium weight loss program.

You'll discover how to keep those pounds off for the rest of your born days.

You can lower your cholesterol.

EXERCISE! EXERCISE! EXERCISE!

Surprise! You'll have more energy. You'll be slimmer. Less baggage to drag around.

Your everyday nutritious eating will give you more pep.

Exercise pumps you up with extra oxygen.

You'll be happier with your beautiful bod, you babe, you.

You'll normalize your life. Never will you have to get twitchy about when and how you'll cheat. You know when your Cheating Day is. No more cheating decisions. Your mind is free. You can write the great American novel or a diet book.

I realize that all this sounds too good to be true, but what can I say? Controlled Cheating has worked for me for thirty-two years. And it can work for everyone. But please see your doctor first.

If you've tried to lose weight and it hasn't worked, maybe it's time you started cheating. Controlled Cheating, with my help. After all, what have you got to lose?

THIS IS NOT A DIET BOOK

"Whoa, Goldberg, I just forked over ten bucks for 220 pages so I could lose this tractor tire hanging around my middle. I need a miracle.

"Now you say Controlled Cheating isn't a diet book. What am I supposed to do with this thing, use it as a door stopper?"

Hold on, pal, *Controlled Cheating* is better than a diet book, it's an eating book. *Controlled Cheating* is also a road map to weight loss, a way-of-life book, a life saver, and a good place to put a wet can of Diet Coke.

DIETS DON'T WORK

Folks go on a diet so that they can get off the diet. Then the hungry dieter starts stuffing it in again. All the lost pounds come back, and probably more.

DIETING IS DUMB . . . but smart people do it.

DIETING IS NOT EASY

Controlled Cheating is not easy either. Controlled Cheating is *easier* because you can cheat. That's it. No secrets. No rattling of magic fried chicken bones. It's just you and that brownie.

Most weight control systems don't allow for the possibility of cheating—Controlled Cheating is based on the certainty of it.

This whole book is based on the only healthy way to lose weight and keep it off; EAT LESS AND EXERCISE MORE.

Controlled Cheating works. Get your tootsies in the starting blocks. We're going to walk to that slim finish line.

Say YES to Controlled Cheating and losing weight and Controlled Cheating will say YES to you.

Think about what you eat every day. Not what you can't eat.

HOW CONTROLLED CHEATING WORKS

As Julius Caesarberg once said: All Controlled Cheating is divided into three parts:

EXERCISE: To lose weight, to keep it off, to lose a size, E-X-E-R-C-I-S-E

EATING PLAN: You will eat plenty of fruits, vegetables, and whole grains; some low-fat poultry, meats, and dairy products; and nutritious foods low in sodium and sugar. The details are coming a few pages down the road in a chapter called "Take My Diet, Please."
You will love it.

CHEATING: You're already an expert.

Now for the details.
1. Set a Goal Weight—consult with your doctor!
2. Follow the Eating Plan for fourteen days or two weeks, whichever is shorter.
3. After the Famished Fortnight, you can cheat for ONE DAY.

4. You can pick any day of the week to cheat.
5. Once you choose your beloved Cheating Day, you cannot change the day.
6. You can cheat one day a week until you reach your Goal Weight.
7. When you reach your Goal Weight, you may CHEAT TWO DAYS, BUT NOT IN A ROW. For instance, you can cheat Wednesday and Saturday, or Thursday and Sunday, or Monday and Thursday. You cannot Cheat Saturday and Sunday, or Wednesday and Thursday. Do I make myself clear? We'll talk about this later.
8. You will then be a slim person.

PICKING THE DAY TO START
YOUR CONTROLLED CHEATING PROGRAM

Monday is the best day to start your diet. How come? I started my diet on a Monday, thirty-two years ago, and I'm such a good guy I want to give you every advantage I had.

Everyone else starts their diets on Mondays, so you'll have lots of grumpy company. Of course, the obvious reason is that everybody hogs it up on the weekends and feels guilty, since they're bursting out of their tight jeans on a Monday morning.

The weekend is the toughest time for us weight losers. Everyone is off work, running to the beach, shopping, or just lying around the house trying to remember some area of the refrigerator that hasn't already been explored.

Social events are mostly on weekends, and who can resist dinner at the home of a great cook or the wedding of your cousin's daughter's niece where the caterer is a sugar sadist?

When you start on a Monday, there are five full days to lose some weight and build your mighty resolve before the critical weekend when you want to stick your whole head in a gallon of rum raisin ice cream and can't.

Anyway, Mondays are rotten! Work begins again, the weekend's over, it always rains on Monday, bills come on Monday, folks are normally in bad moods, and the only good show on television is Monday Night Football.

When you start dieting on Monday, it will be only one of a hundred other miserable things you're doing, and you won't even notice you're eating a plain baked potato with no butter.

CHEATING BEFORE YOU DIET

Okay, you're ready. You've made the biggie, that hard-rock decision. This coming Monday, regardless of what you have to do or how you feel, is D (Diet) Day. Feel better already? You bet. No more horsing around, no more waiting until after Groundhog Day, or after that Kansas City Royals–New York Yankees doubleheader so that you can stuff down the juicy hot dogs with horseradish, mustard, and cold foamy root beer.

From now until *the* Monday, eat what you want, but in moderation. Don't make those first two weeks any harder than they are already. This is the time, just before your diet starts, to starting eating the way a thin person eats. After all, that's what you're going to be from now on. Don't eat like a loco grizzly bear who has to put on an extra layer of suet to keep warm through the winter. Or like a condemned man getting that final meal on earth before Pat O'Brien, as the priest, comes in to walk you down that last mile.

That's the joy of Controlled Cheating, a new, thin life where you don't have to give up anything, where all the foods you love the most will be ready and waiting for you every single week.

Some of the most helpful parts of my program are not usually mentioned in diet books. But dieting is a permanent part of my life. I want it to sing along in harmony with other things that are important to me. I couldn't diet successfully without laughter.

THE D (DIET) DAY WAKE-UP CALL

The clock radio clicks on, playing "Junk Food Junkie," jolting you back from a yummy dream of climbing up a mountain of fresh ripe strawberries on a shortcake ladder while you're carrying a bag of whipped cream.

Sleep catches you with all your defenses down. At no time in your dieting life are you more vulnerable. Rub the sleep from your eyes, slap a smile on your face, and leap out of bed. Today is THE DAY.

You scream, "Oh God, no! It's Monday and I have to start my Controlled Cheating Diet Program that some guy named Goldberg says has worked for him over thirty years and will work for me. If he's such a hotshot dieter, let him do it for me. I'll start tomorrow—maybe."

Right there, right at that instant, stop that thought and replace it with a positive proclamation starting your diet today. That's NOW, not tomorrow, or next week. This is called Positive Waking Up. Like everyone else, I have negative, dumb thoughts when I wake up. I've discovered that if I can substitute good, positive vibrations shooting through my brain for the first fifteen minutes, I have the rest of the day made.

You can use this system, too. It takes practice, but soon it will come automatically. What a difference it will make in your life. Think about the food hangovers, volcano-hot heartburn, and the Snickers-stained shirts you'll never have again.

When you've got your mind giggling, tap dance into the bathroom and, with plenty of sweet toothpaste, give your teeth the workout of their lives. While you're riding the Crest, start thinking about fourteen days from now and the good eats you're going to choose for your Cheating Day. See, right away you can look forward to a pot of gold, or at least pasta, at the end of the rainbow.

I want you to look forward to your diet meals, too. We all know how much fun eating is. Make your breakfast, lunch, dinner, and snacks, big, happy events. You might even blow up a few balloons. Plus, if you eat very slooooooowly, the fun of eating will go on and on.

FIRST DAY

Don't start feeling sorry for yourself, ever. Especially not on this crucial first day. So you don't get to eat a hunk of creamy cheesecake. So what! You've only got to wait for a couple of weeks and you can have nine pieces of creamy cheesecake—plus a glass of cream, if you want.

I know, I know, you're so hungry you're about to start licking the plaster off the walls. Hey, I'm right with you all the way. After thirty-two years, I still get as hungry on Non-Cheating Days as I did the first day I started. YOU CAN DO IT. If I, Fats Goldberg, foodaholic, human garbage can, and all-around weak person, can do it, you sure can. Why? Because we can look at that beautiful horizon and eyeball your gorgeous Cheating Day.

Carry this book along with you on the first day and every day for the next two weeks. *Really* learn what you can and cannot eat, and, just as important, the portion sizes. Make notes in it, draw funny faces, put your homeroom number in the front. Read it while you're eating. If you're lucky, maybe a few crumbs will fall in the pages. Later in the day you can lick your finger, pick up the crumbs, and have an evening snack.

Your first Diet Day is about over. Congratulations, you soon-to-be-thin person. I know you've stuck to the diet. Hooray! Only thirteen more days until Broadway, your first Cheating Day.

Tomorrow morning you'll get up, hop on the scale, and maybe see some results from today. Don't get twitchy if there is no movement on the scale right away. We lose weight in stair steps, not in a perfect slide. That stupid needle might not move right away, especially at the beginning, and then *pow,* you'll drop a whole load of pounds all at once—and you'll keep dropping.

As I tuck you in, and you snuggle down for an indigestion-free sleep, before I tiptoe out, I must scream that under no circumstances are you to take any diet pills or any over-the-counter appetite depressants or diet aids. Save your money for an extra dessert on a Cheating Day; it'll do you more good.

THIRTEEN IS YOUR LUCKY NUMBER

Congrats, you've gotten through the most awful day and night of your Controlled Cheating life. Now what's thirteen more Diet Days to a diet professional like you? But wait, don't break your arm patting yourself on the back. (It's all right to give yourself a few hugs, though.)

I know you can sail through the weekdays of dieting like a swift breeze. After all, you've got your career, or there's the fun of housework, or whatever you do Monday through Friday. The stickler is the weekend. You must double your determination on Saturday and Sunday. When you get down to it, there are only four measly days you have to worry about. Keeping busy is the answer. The devil finds Peanut M&M's for idle hands.

Here are some Weekend Wonders that I've used:
1. Exercise MORE!
2. Make a big list of activities for each day: Clean out the garage; play golf, tennis, stickball, or all three; go shopping (stay out of supermarkets unless accompanied by a friend or relative with a strong pair of handcuffs); or go to a museum. I especially like museums because there are no refreshment stands and you can meet a fancy, smart person.
3. Stuff your ice box with big bowls of cut-up vegetables and fruits, such as carrots, celery, tomatoes, cauliflower, and other crunchies. On Diet Days I like foods that require heavy chewing and make plenty of noise. You can fake yourself out that you're having huge meals, plus filling your tummy with good nutrition at the same time.
4. If you are going out to dinner or a hot party, eat some of those low-calorie foods before leaving home. They'll take the edge off your appetite. Then you won't leap into the middle of the goody table or dump the bread and butter basket on your head.

5. You cannot drink alcoholic beverages during the first fourteen days. Stick to plain tap water, the chic sparkling water with a spritz of lime, coffee and tea (no sugar or cream, please), or sugar-free soda with lots of ice.

6. Go see *Grease*, *Sugar Babies*, or a Meatloaf concert.

GOLDBERG'S FIVE-POUNDER

No, this isn't the biggest burger McDonald's ever made, with pickles, onions, mustard, and ketchup. This is my system for setting your Goal Weight, getting to it, and sticking to it.

You know what your ideal weight is, or what you want it to be. Once you've set your Goal Weight, think of it as divided into five-pound bites. When you've chewed away the first Five-Pounder, go for another Five-Pounder and then all the weight down. If you're more than twenty-five pounds overweight, your ultimate goal may seem impossible, but taking it in five-pound bites will give you reachable, intermediate successes that will spur you on to the next Five-Pounder. Soon all the fives you subtract will add up to your true goal!

You might say, "Hey Goldberg, I have to lose fifty-five pounds. Five measly pounds is nothing."

If you don't think five pounds is much weight, I want you to take the Goldberg's Supermarket Schlep Test. Here's how:

Go into your local grocery store and pick up a five-pound bag of potatoes and hoist it over your head. That's the weight you have just taken off your poor sagging bones. You might get some funny looks from the blue-haired ladies thumping watermelons, but just smile triumphantly.

After you lose another five, go back and lift ten pounds over your head. The same ladies will probably still be there. If they call the manager, run to the detergent department and hide. Keep testing with every five-pound loss until you think you might get a hernia.

Everything you do for yourself takes time. It took a long

time to put on that fat, and there is no way you're going to lose it overnight. That's why Controlled Cheating works. You'll only have to diet for two short weeks at the start; then every week after that, you'll be able to eat as much as you want of whatever you want for a whole day. French-fried everything, here I come!

YOUR POWER, *NOT* WILL POWER

Hey Will Power, hey Wilma Power, come out, come out, wherever you are. You're not there? How come? Everyone says you have to have something called "willpower" to lose and keep off weight. Forget it. There's no such thing. If there were, I would have found it. I've been looking for that son of a gun in every place I've seen the word "diet."

Willpower is a cop-out. It's probably the most overused, dumb expression ever invented. I should know. I conned myself for twenty-five years saying "I don't have any willpower." Like I could go to the Quik Trip and pick up a pint from the freezer.

No blinding ray of light will shoot down from parting fat clouds to give you will power.

You're sitting at the kitchen table. A big bowl of soft French vanilla ice cream with hot fudge and almonds is in front of you. That bowl is screaming at you to grab a tablespoon and bless your mouth with indescribable joy.

It all boils down to whether you're going to bury your face in that ice cream or not. No magic will power is going to hold your quivering shoulders and shout a great big "NO!"

The only power we have is inside ourselves. There's no Goldberg Power. There's no President "Broccoli" Bush power.

You have to do it. The strongest power you'll ever have is YOUR POWER and your sense of humor.

GOLDBERG POWER?

If I, weak Fats Goldberg, can lose 175 pounds and keep it off for thirty-two years, then you, frustrated person, or anyone else who ever gnawed on a carrot trying to lose a few ounces, can lose weight and keep it off. I guarantee it.

Let's you and I pull up a couple of ice cream chairs and talk about Goldberg Power. There's no such power. I'm not Superman. What I am is a fat man disguised as a thin man. (I don't have the shoulders to be Superman and I used to need about four times the space of a phone booth just to put on my boxer shorts.)

What's Goldberg Power? Very simply it's DO IT! DO IT! DO IT!

Aren't you getting tired of reading diet books, fantasizing about being slim and good-looking with enough energy to dance all night and run a five-mile race in the morning?

For me, and now for you, too, the time for talking is over. Now is the time to act. First, there is no such thing as a perfect time for you to start dieting. The time to start is now.

Smarts, discipline, laughs, slimness, and everything else you'll ever have or want are inside that beautiful body of yours. No one but YOU can make you lose weight and keep it off. The only way to release the tremendous power you have is to start tapping your great ocean of inner resources. Once your strengths start gushing to the surface, a Texas oil well will look like a drop in the bucket.

Losing weight and keeping it off is a difficult, no fun business. At different times for the rest of your Controlled Cheating life, every ounce of guts you can muster will help you not to eat that Twinkie.

I'm going to be with you every step of the way because I've already gone down that Yellow Mozzarella Brick Road to the Emerald City. What all this boils down to is whether or not you're going to eat that slab of ribs when you shouldn't.

Everything starts with *YOU*!

WHY CONTROLLED CHEATING WORKS

Controlled Cheating works because you, me, and the rest of the world can't eat that much.

When I started Controlled Cheating, I never exactly knew why I was losing weight and eating everything I craved on my Cheating Days.

Sure I was reducing the fat at a steady slide. Old Fats was exercising and eating normal portions of healthy foods. Then, on my Cheating Days, I was stuffing in the grease, dough, and sugar. But how did it really work?

After I dropped a ton, flabby folks started coming up and whispering how they wanted to lose some weight. I never told anyone exactly how I did it because I thought with such a crazy diet, they'd shove me in The Home For The Distraught.

Ten years ago in Kansas City, the Parelman family pinned me against the kitchen sink and insisted that I tell them how I lost all the suet. This was the first time I told anyone the complete program. The whole family lost weight and all of them are still healthy and slim.

The biggest surprise of my life was making up the sample

Cheating Days. Looking at the calorie totals solved The Mystery of Controlled Cheating.

First the facts:
- You have to eat 3500 calories to gain a pound.
- You have to burn 3500 calories to lose a pound.

This is true for every human being regardless of weight, sex, or age.

Get out your pencils and paper.

The 1200 calorie eating plan I'm going to talk about is an average for both women and men.

To maintain her weight, an average woman needs 1800 to 2000 calories per day. A man needs 2400 to 2700 calories per day.

Because our individual calorie needs are so different, I suggest you see your doctor about how many calories YOU need to lose weight safely.

1. Suppose for six days you eat about 1500 calories, which is a healthy calorie count for losing weight.
2. Multiply by six and you eat 9000 calories in six days.
3. On your Cheating Day, you eat about 5000 calories, which is a lot for any fatty.
4. You've eaten 14,000 calories for the week.
5. Divide by seven days, and you're averaging 2000 calories daily.
6. Figuring you're burning at least 500 or 600 calories a day with your exercise program and other physical messing around, you're averaging about 1500 calories a day.
7. At 1500 calories, you're losing weight. Simple, huh? All right, gang, what have we learned today?

THE REASON WHY CONTROLLED CHEATING WORKS IS BECAUSE HUMAN BEINGS CANNOT EAT THAT MUCH.

You think you can. Which is why Controlled Cheating is successful and fun.

You must have a regular exercise program. EXERCISE BURNS CALORIES. So stop complaining about moving your tush.

If you don't have a consistent exercise program, Controlled Cheating WILL NOT WORK.

Yeah, yeah, I've heard it all before. Everybody thinks they can easily eat ten or fifteen thousand calories on their Cheating Day. I can't, you can't, and they can't.

Ma and Pa were right. Our eyes are bigger than our stomachs.

TAKE MY DIET, PLEASE

Yesiree, you can take my eating plan, get slim, stay healthy, eat good food, and become beautiful (or handsome).

My diet is great for me and other folks who have used it. But depending on your age, sex, build, and how much exercise you do, your body may have special needs—consult your doctor.

Food alone can't make you vigorous and sparkly. But good eating habits can improve your health and help keep you healthy.

A good diet consists of fruits, vegetables, whole grains, lean meat, poultry, fish, and low-fat dairy products. The Goldberg Eating Plan is high in nutrients and low in fat, sugar, salt, and cholesterol.

Hold on now. No one superfood supplies all the essential nutrients you need. You have to eat a variety from every food group daily. Mix your favorite foods with new stuff. Dining on the same eats all the time is boring and no fun. You could blow the whole Controlled Cheating program because you've eaten so many carrots that your skin is neon orange.

Don't even think of this as a diet. *Diet* is a nasty four-letter word. Controlled Cheating is a lifetime eating plan. Experiment. Use your food imagination. Try new foods. Get out of the same old monotonous ruts.

So you ask, "What's the gimmick?" No gimmick. You only have to make the right food choices.

1. Eat a variety of foods
2. Eat plenty of starches and fiber
3. Eat plenty of vegetables, fruits, and grain products
4. Phooey on fats
5. Cease with the sugar
6. Halt the salt
7. Allay the alcohol
8. Save all the grease, dough, sugar, salt, and alcohol for your Cheating Days

THE GOLDBERG EATING PLAN

"So Goldberg, what am I going to eat on the Famished Fortnight to lose weight before I get to that Cheating Day?"

Relax, pal. You're never going to be famished if I have anything to say about it. I've found a terrific eating plan. Believe it or not, it came from the United States Department of Agriculture. Finally, you're going to get something for your taxes. The booklet is titled: "Nutrition and Your Health: Dietary Guidelines for Americans: Eat a Variety of Foods." This is only one of a big bunch of dynamite nutrition books and cookbooks the feds publish. Stop by a government bookstore or call 1-800-735-8004. That is the Government Information Line, and they'll tell you how to get a catalog of publications.

This eating plan will let you pick what *you* want to eat. It's not one of those horrible rigid diet programs that tells you exactly what you have to eat at every meal. I hate that. Maybe I don't want to eat a quarter of a honeydew for breakfast on Tuesday. Variety is the spice that keeps this program fun and interesting.

This is a nutritionally sound eating plan that you can live with for the rest of your life. For some of us, dieting has to become a way of life, for our whole lives, not just a two-week fling with being famished and then back to the binge. There are no calories to count and no miraculous promises. Just lots to eat from a huge range of good, healthy food. You will never be denied nutritious food.

The Goldberg Eating Plan (I put my name in there because I pay taxes too) has seven food groups:

FOOD GROUPS	SUGGESTED DAILY SERVINGS
1. Breads, Cereals, Rice, and Pasta	6–11 servings
2. Vegetables	3 or more servings
3. Fruits	2 or more servings
4. Meat, Poultry, Fish, Dry Beans and Peas, Eggs, and Nuts	2–3 servings
5. Milk, Cheese, and Yogurt	2–3 servings
6. Fats and Oils	5–7 teaspoons
7. Sweets and Alcoholic Beverages	0 servings

- Cut way down on fats. Don't eat any sweets or drink any alcoholic beverages except on Cheating Days.
- Choose foods daily from each of the first five groups.
- Include different foods from within the groups.
- Have at least the smaller number of servings suggested from each group.

The amount of food you need depends on your age, sex, physical condition, and how much exercise you do. But even if you're a 250-pound marathon runner, don't exceed the maximum suggested servings of any food group.

Remember there is no one food that supplies all the essential nutrients in the amounts you need. So it's important you eat several types of food from each group each day.

Fats, sweets, and alcoholic beverages provide few vitamins and minerals, but they do give you plenty of empty calories. Wait for your Cheating Day.

The Goldberg Eating Plan is a lifetime eating plan. You will learn how to eat for your beautiful body. When you've slogged through the first fourteen days of no-cheating eating, you'll be right on the royal road to your goal. What you accomplish after these first two weeks may possibly be more satisfying than anything you've ever done before. You're a champ!

I'll be waiting for you with a twenty-five-pound bag of caramel corn at the finish line.

Use the following chart as your eating guide. Vary your diet, be creative, but never eat more than the maximum serving.

WHAT TO EAT AND HOW MUCH

FOOD GROUP	SUGGESTED DAILY SERVINGS	WHAT COUNTS AS A SERVING?
BREADS, CEREALS, RICE, AND PASTA • Whole grain • Enriched	6–11 Include in the several servings a day a variety of grain products such as wheat, rice, oats, and corn	• 1 slice of bread • ½ hamburger bun, English muffin, or bagel • a small roll, biscuit, or muffin • 3 to 4 small or 2 large crackers • ½ cup cooked cereal, rice, or pasta • 1 ounce dry, ready-to-eat breakfast cereal

EXAMPLES (keep to these and you won't go wrong)
WHOLE GRAIN: Bagels (water), bread sticks, buckwheat groats, bulgur, corn tortillas, graham crackers, matzo, oatmeal, popcorn, pumpernickel bread, ready-to-eat cereals (not presweetened), rye crackers, whole wheat bread and rolls, whole wheat crackers, whole wheat pasta, whole wheat cereals
ENRICHED: Bagels (water), biscuits, corn bread, corn muffins, cornmeal, crackers (low fat), English muffins, farina, French bread, grits, hamburger rolls, hot dog buns, Italian bread, macaroni, muffins, noodles, pasta, ready-to-eat cereals (not presweetened), rice

VEGETABLES
- Dark-green leafy
- Deep yellow
- Dry beans and peas (legumes)
- Starchy
- Other Vegetables

3 or more
Include all types regularly; eat dark-green leafy vegetables, legumes, unsalted vegetable juices, and starchy vegetables such as potatoes and corn several times a week

- ½ cup of chopped raw or cooked vegetables
- 1 cup of leafy raw vegetables such as lettuce or spinach
- count ½ cup of cooked dry beans or peas as a serving of vegetables or as 1 ounce of the meat group

EXAMPLES
DARK-GREEN LEAFY: Beet greens, broccoli, chard, chicory, collard greens, dandelion greens, endive, escarole, kale, mustard greens, romaine lettuce, spinach, turnip greens, watercress
DEEP YELLOW: Carrots, pumpkin, sweet potato, winter squash
STARCHY: Corn, green peas, hominy, lima beans, potato, rutabaga
LEGUMES: Black beans, black-eyed peas, chickpeas (garbanzos), kidney beans, lentils, lima beans (mature), mung beans, navy beans, pinto beans, split peas
OTHER VEGETABLES: Artichoke, asparagus, bean and alfalfa sprouts, beets, brussels sprouts, cabbage, cauliflower, celery, Chinese cabbage, cucumber, eggplant, green beans, green pepper, lettuce, mushrooms, okra, onions (mature and green), radishes, summer squash, tomato, turnip, vegetable juices, zucchini

---

FRUITS
- Citrus, melon, berries
- Other fruits

2 or more
Choose fruits as desserts and fruit juices as beverages

- a whole fruit such as a medium apple, banana, or orange
- a grapefruit half
- a melon wedge
- ¾ cup of juice
- ½ cup of berries or diced fruit
- ½ cooked or canned fruit (no sugar added)
- ¼ cup dried fruit
Always try to eat fresh fruits, including at least one citrus a day

EXAMPLES
CITRUS, MELONS, AND BERRIES: Blueberries, cantaloupe, citrus juices, cranberries, grapefruit, honeydew melon, kiwi fruit, lemon, orange, raspberries, strawberries, tangerine, watermelon
OTHER FRUITS: Apple, apricot, banana, cherries, dates, figs, fruit juices, grapes, guava, mango, nectarine, papaya, peach, pear, pineapple, plantain, plum, pomegranate, prunes, raisins

LEAN MEAT,	2–3	Amounts should total 6 oz. of
POULTRY,	6 oz. of cooked	cooked lean meat, poultry
FISH, EGGS,	lean beef or	(without skin), or fish a day. A
DRY BEANS	chicken without	serving of meat the size and
AND PEAS	skin provides	thickness of the palm of a
	about the equiva-	woman's hand is about 3–5 oz.
	lent of 3 teaspoons	and a man's 5–7 oz. Count 1
	of fat—count this	egg or ½ cup cooked beans as 1
	toward your daily	oz. of meat.
	fats and oils total	
	(see below)	

EXAMPLES

Poultry without skin—all kinds; Fish—all kinds (tuna and other canned fish should be packed in water); Shellfish—all kinds

LEAN CUTS OF MEAT WITH FAT TRIMMED: Beef—round, sirloin, chuck, loin, brisket, lean ground beef; Lamb—leg, arm, loin, rib; Pork—tenderloin, leg (fresh), shoulder (arm or picnic); Veal—all trimmed cuts; Eggs; Legumes (see above under "vegetables")

MILK,	2–3 (3 for teens)	•1 cup of milk
CHEESE,		•8 oz. of fat-free or low-fat
AND		yogurt (1 cup)
YOGURT		•1½ oz. of natural cheese

EXAMPLES

LOWFAT MILK PRODUCTS: Buttermilk, cheese (labeled 2–6 grams of fat per ounce), evaporated or dry low-fat milk, frozen yogurt (low-fat or no fat), ice milk, milk (1% or skim), soft cheeses (*low-fat* cottage, farmer, pot, Parmesan, feta, skim mozzarella, or ricotta), yogurt

---

FATS AND	5–7 teaspoons
OILS	Use for cooking
	and salad dressings

EXAMPLES

CHOOSE: Unsaturated vegetable oils: corn, olive, peanut, rapeseed (canola), safflower, sesame, soybean; Salad dressings, margarine, or shortening made from the unsaturated fats listed above: liquid, tub, stick or diet

USE ONLY ON CHEATING DAYS: Butter, coconut oil, palm oil, palm kernel oil, lard, bacon fat, margarine or shortening made from saturated fats listed above

---

That's *what* you eat. *How* you eat it is up to you. But as you might guess, I've got a few suggestions on the topic:

EAT BREAKFAST LIKE A QUEEN OR KING

Why and how you should put on the feed bag in the morning:

- You'll quick-start your heart.
- You're opening those baby blues after an eight-hour fast.
- The tummy is empty. You need fuel to fill up the tank.
- Even if you're like Dracula in the early sunlight, try to eat something in the hour or two after getting up.
- Gnaw on a piece of fruit or a glass of unsweetened juice.
- Slurp up plenty of proteins, like a bowl of Grape Nuts and skim milk. Maybe even slice a banana on top. This is my favorite.
- For instant energizers, eat some of those complex carbohydrates like whole-grain breads, cereals, muffins, bagels, vegetables, and fruit.
- Skipping breakfast will drive you crazy with hunger and you might blow your Diet Day on lunch or dinner.
- I know you don't give a doughnut hole, but breakfast and brunch are my favorite meals.

NIBBLING, NOSHING, SNACKING, AND GRAZING

Three squares are out . . . little meals are in.
How come?

- Nibbling is healthier. Our bodies are made for small meals.
- Minimeals are easier to digest.
- The food goes right to work. It doesn't have time to be stored as fat.
- You don't get so hungry or feel deprived.
- You won't have to wait so long to eat. Something good is right around the corner in the refrigerator door.

- Our food fantasies are minutes away.
- Lots of chewing all day long. Your wisdom teeth, if you have any, won't get cobwebs.
- BUT you have to choose nutritious and healthy noshing, not those greasy, sugary, salty snacks in little cellophane bags.
- *You'll feel perpetually peppy.*

GOLDBERG'S HEALTHY SNACKS, BREAKS, HUNGER STOPPERS, OR ANYTIME YOU GET TWITCHY

- Crunch and munch on: raw veggies, fresh fruits, hot-air popcorn, rice cakes, unsalted pretzels, a bagel, low-fat crackers, whole-wheat pita bread.
- Slurp and sip on: skim milk, no-fat yogurt (slice in some fruits or vegetables; add spices like cinnamon, or a few raisins).
- Drink water. Maybe put in a squeeze of lemon or lime. Drink salt-free veggie juices.
- Take a walk.
- Grab your sweetie pie and do some hugging and kissing. (It doesn't even have to be your sweetie pie.)
- Cut, slice, or chop all sorts of healthy snacks and leave them in your fridge for a quick nosh.
- Use your own wonderful food imagination and invent some healthy nibbling. If you come up with something that tastes and feels like apple pie a la mode with zero calories, let me know.

NUTRIENTS: THE LOWDOWN

WHAT ARE THEY?
WHO ARE THEY?
HOW ARE THEY?
FINE, THANK YOU.

Fasten your seat belts. This could be a bumpy ride.

There are six nutrients: carbohydrates, fats, proteins, vitamins, minerals, and water.

CARBOHYDRATES

They include starches, sugars, and dietary fiber. Starch and sugar supply the body with energy. Dietary fiber provides bulk to the diet, which helps to clean you out.

Carbohydrates have four calories per gram—the same calories as protein and *less than half* the calories of fat.

There are two kinds of carbohydrates: complex and simple. Our dear Mother Nature packaged simple and complex carbohydrates in foods like oranges, apples, corn, wheat, and milk.

Refined or processed carbohydrates are found in cookies, cakes, and pies. They're yummy, but save them for your Cheating Day.

COMPLEX CARBOHYDRATES: Complex carbohydrates are the starches and fiber found in plants.

HOT NEWS ABOUT STARCH AND FIBER: The major sources of energy are carbohydrates and fats. So, dear dieter, when we cut down on fat, we need to eat *more* starchy foods. Unlike sugars and sweets, starchy foods pour in the vitamins and minerals as well as energy.

Since complex carbohydrates have only four calories per gram, while fat provides nine calories per gram, if you eat more starchy fiber foods, you can fill up that tummy with fewer calories.

FUN WITH FIBER: Most of us don't eat enough fiber. Dietary fiber—a part of plant foods—is in whole grain breads and cereals, dried beans and peas, vegetables, and fruits. We have to eat a variety of these fiber-rich foods because they differ in the kinds of fiber they contain.

Eating foods with fiber is important for proper bowel function and can reduce symptoms of chronic constipation, diverticular disease, and hemorrhoids. Populations like ours with diets low in dietary fiber and complex carbohydrates, and high in fat, especially saturated fat, tend to have more heart disease, obesity, and some cancers. Just how dietary fiber is involved isn't very clear.

Some of the benefit from a higher fiber diet may be from the food that provides the fiber, not from fiber alone. It's best to get fiber from foods rather than from supplements. In addition, too much from supplements is associated with greater risk for intestinal problems and lower absorption of some minerals.

Now here's the right stuff you should be eating in the sensational complex-carbohydrate food department:

- Fresh fruits and raw vegetables
- Whole-grain everything: wheat, corn, rice, bread, cereals, and pasta
- Legumes: dried beans and peas
- The National Cancer Institute says we should eat 20–30 grams of fiber a day.
- A plain baked potato with the skin has over four grams of fiber and no fat, plus you're getting 50 percent of the vitamin C you need daily.
- Drink lots of water.
- Complex carbohydrates taste good, with lots of crunching and chewing. Great aerobics for the mouth.
- Fiber reduces the symptoms of constipation and keeps your insides healthy.
- Don't go overboard eating fiber—thirty-five grams is maximum. Too much could stop the absorption of vitamins and minerals.
- One slice of 100 percent whole wheat bread has three times the fiber of one slice of white bread.
- AND with complex carbohydrates, YOU'RE ALWAYS FULL. Wowee.

SIMPLE CARBOHYDRATES: Simple carbohydrates are sugars, such as table sugar (sucrose), honey, corn syrup, molasses. They provide "empty" calories—that's to say, they give you the energy without the nutrition.

PHOOEY ON FATS AND
CHUCK THE CHOLESTEROL

FAT: Fat supplies nine calories per gram, more than twice the number provided by carbohydrates or protein. But fat also helps our absorption of vitamins, and small amounts of fat are necessary for normal body function.

There are three kinds of fats: saturated, polyunsaturated, and monounsaturated. A mixture of all three in varying amounts is in most of our food.

SATURATED FAT: This baby is found in greatest amounts in meat, poultry, and whole-milk dairy products. Stinky saturated fats are also found in vegetable oils like coconut, palm kernel, and palm oils. SATURATED FAT RAISES BLOOD CHOLESTEROL MORE THAN ANYTHING ELSE IN THE DIET.

UNSATURATED FATS: You should substitute these for saturated fats in your diet: *POLYUNSATURATED FATS* are found in plant products like safflower, sunflower, corn, soybean, and cottonseed oils; nuts and seeds; and fatty fish. *MONOUNSATURATED FATS* are primarily found in olive oil and canola oil.

CHOLESTEROL is a fat-like, waxy substance, and is found in foods of animal origin: high-fat foods like hot dogs and cheddar cheese, and low-fat foods like liver and other organ meats.

- A daily intake of less than 300 mg of cholesterol is good.
- A 3 oz. piece of meat, fish, or poultry has 60-90 mg of cholesterol; one egg yolk contains about 270 mg, and a 3 oz. piece of liver has about 390 mg.

Okay—what's *your* cholesterol count? Through the wonders of modern medicine, your doctor can tell you in a flash.

The medical guys recently set guidelines for blood cholesterol levels. They say that a total cholesterol level of less than 200 mg/dl is desirable for adults—above 200 mg/dl the risk of coronary heart disease increases. Take a peek at the following:

200 mg/dl or less—GOOD
200–240 mg/dl—BORDERLINE
240 mg/dl and above—HIGH

HYDROGENATED FATS: These fats and oils are changed from their natural liquid form to become solid to increase shelf life—examples are most margarines and shortenings. They may be partially or almost completely hydrogenated oils: they resemble saturated fats, and that means you want to avoid them. Many margarines contain partially hydrogenated oils and may be okay if they contain twice as much polyunsaturated fat as saturated fat. Read those interesting labels.

HOW TO CUT BACK ON SATURATED FATS AND CHOLESTEROL:
- Choose poultry, fish, and lean meats. Take the skin from chicken and trim the fat from meat.
- Drink skim milk or 1% milk.
- Use tub margarine or liquid vegetable oils that are high in unsaturated fat like safflower, corn, and olive oil, instead of butter, lard, and hydrogenated vegetable shortening, which are high in saturated fat.
- Cut down on commercially prepared and processed foods made with saturated fats and oils.

PROTEINS

Proteins are one of the three nutrients that supply energy or calories to our beautiful bodies. Protein provides four calories per gram, which again is half the calories of fat.

Proteins are essential for building, maintaining, repairing, and replacing tissues in the heart, brain, muscles, bones, skin, and blood.

Proteins are in every living cell.

We only need about six ounces of protein food daily—foods such as poultry, fish, lean meats, low-fat dairy products, and legumes.

Our bodies need protein foods every day. We can't store proteins. The older we get, the less protein we need.

If we eat more protein than we need, it will turn to fat.

VITAMINS

Vitamins are essential to life.

They are organic substances needed by the body in very small amounts, about an eighth of a teaspoon a day. They don't supply energy, but they help release energy from carbohydrates, fats, and proteins. Vitamins also help in other chemical reactions in your body.

MINERALS

Minerals are also needed in small amounts and do not supply energy. They are used to build strong bones and teeth, and to make hemoglobin in red blood cells. Minerals help maintain body fluids and help in other chemical reactions in the body. They are just as important as vitamins.

The only pill I pop in my mouth is one of those one-a-day vitamin and mineral supplements as a little health insurance. The one I take does not exceed 100 percent of the recommended daily allowance of any vitamin or mineral.

Before you douse yourself with megadoses of vitamins and minerals, see your doctor.

WATER

Water is often called the "forgotten nutrient." It is needed to replace body water lost in urine and sweat. Good old water helps transport nutrients and remove wastes, and keeps our body temperature okay.

Water is so important to me, that I give it a whole chapter down the river. So keep your cup ready and your faucet running.

WHAT ABOUT CALORIES?

A calorie is a measure of the energy supplied by food when it is used by the body. Our bodies need energy to perform work. The nutrients that supply calories (energy) are carbohydrates, fat, and protein. The alcohol in beer, wine, and hard liquor also supplies calories.

COOL IT ON THE SUGAR

What's sugar?

Most folks figure that "sugar" means white table sugar. But sugar means all forms of sweeteners, including white sugar (sucrose), brown sugar, raw sugar, glucose (dextrose), fructose, maltose, lactose, high fructose corn syrup, honey, corn sweetener, syrup, fruit juice concentrate, and molasses. Read those food labels. A food is likely to be high in sugars if its ingredient list shows one of the above first or second or if it shows several of them.

SUGAR? WHAT COMES NATURALLY? Most fruits and some vegetables contain sugars such as glucose, fructose, and sucrose. Another sugar, lactose, is found in milk and milk products. Legumes and cereals contain small amounts of maltose. Besides sugars, these foods provide needed vitamins and minerals. Remember, we've already talked about complex carbohydrates.

WHAT'S ADDED? Sugars are added to foods during processing, making foods in the home, or at the table. Listen to this: sugar is used more in food processing than any other additive.

SUGAR AND YOUR HEALTH. Sugar gives us energy (calories) but few nutrients. Being overweight results from stuffing in too many calories. Cutting back on added sugars is a good way to reduce calories—without reducing nutrients. Too much sugar has not been shown to cause diabetes or heart disease, but being fat IS associated with a greater risk of both of these disorders. Again, eat those complex carbohydrates and cut back on simple carbohydrates.

WHAT ABOUT ARTIFICIAL SWEETENERS? You don't need artificial sweeteners to reduce sugars in your diet.

HALT THE SALT

WHAT'S SODIUM? Sodium is a mineral that shows up naturally in some foods and is added to many foods and drinks. A lot of sodium in our diet comes from table salt. One teaspoon of salt has about two thousand milligrams of sodium. Whoa!

HOW MUCH SODIUM DO I NEED? Some sodium is good for your health. But you need very little. A safe range of sodium intake per day is about one thousand to three thousand milligrams for adults. This is way below what we eat now.

WHERE IS SODIUM IN MY DIET? Use salt sparingly, if at all, in cooking and at the table. When planning meals, consider that:

- fresh and plain frozen vegetables prepared without salt are lower in sodium than canned ones
- cereals, pasta, and rice cooked without salt are lower in sodium than ready-to-eat cereals
- milk and yogurt are lower in sodium than most cheeses
- fresh meat, poultry, and fish are lower in sodium than most canned and processed counterparts

Use salted snacks, such as chips, crackers, pretzels, and nuts, sparingly.

Check labels for the amount of sodium in foods. Choose those lower in sodium most of the time.

HOT NEWS FOR SALT LOVERS! We were not born with a taste for salt. We *learned* it. This means we can unlearn it by cutting the amount of salt in our diet. Studies show that folks who gradually reduce the amount of salt they eat lose their desire for the salty taste.

THROW THAT SALT SHAKER OUT!

What about salt substitutes? Please ask your doctor.

DRINKING

1947 was a really big year. I was thirteen years old and weighed 240 pounds. At my Bar Mitzvah, I was presented with nine billfolds and ten belts (none of them fit because the givers, of course, underestimated the girth of the thirteen-year-old kid), and I saw a movie that changed my life. The movie was *The Lost Weekend* with Ray Milland and Jane Wyman. Ray got an Academy Award and Jane got Ronald Reagan. Billy Wilder directed and co-wrote.

Don't miss it when it comes on the Late Show. It's the story of an alcoholic writer and his plunge into the depths of sickness, poverty, and hallucinations. And those are only the happy parts.

When I walked out of that movie, I was in a daze. *The Lost Weekend* literally cured my drinking problem before I ever tasted hard liquor. I didn't realize it at the time, though.

The first time I ever drank hard whiskey was in September 1954, in the hot, humid basement of the Zeta Beta Tau fraternity house at the University of Missouri. I got loaded. Boy, did I have a great time for about fifty-seven minutes. Then I stumbled upstairs and had my head in the wash basin for the next two days.

Getting roaring drunk was a Saturday night ritual for about two months. I'd start slow and end up swigging out of the bottle. Then I'd spend the rest of Saturday night and all day Sunday in the third stall of the toilet.

One of the reasons I drank was to give me enough courage to try to "make out" with a little A E Phi cutie I was lavaliered to. You got it. This didn't work either. We'd walk back to her sorority house, go up the stairs to the door, and

I'd get ready for action. She'd stop. I'd make my move. Nothing. A little peck on my pouty lips and she'd bolt.

One Saturday night we were sitting there in the basement with the rest of the gang. Everything was as usual; one bottle of scotch, two dirty water glasses, and my little sweetie.

I looked at that jug of whiskey and I said to myself, "This stuff tastes horrible. What am I doing? It tastes awful, I get sick as a dog, and I don't make out anyway." That's when I decided not to drink anymore. It's been about 30 years now since I've even had a taste of whiskey.

Liquor tasted to me like medicine. I was used to soda, ice cream malts, and sweet things. Drinking was stupid for me, for two reasons. I sure wasn't enjoying the taste, and I had terminal nausea and hangovers. Let me tell you when a 300-pounder has a hangover, that's a severe problem.

What other folks do is fine with me. I can sit in bars, go to parties or anywhere else where there's drinking, and have tomato juice, diet soda, or plain water.

Getting down to the nitty-gritty, I have enough problems with food without bringing in other stuff.

GOLDBERG'S SALOON

What *do* you order if everyone else is sitting around the Dew Drop Inn? There are cocktails you can make any number of ways. Some of them are:

Diet soda with lemon; regular soda "on the rocks"; plain tomato juice (also known as a "Virgin Mary"); plain orange juice (never heard of a clever name for this one—maybe it should be called a "Virgin Driver"); plain club soda, "straight up"; or, of course, the elegant imported waters in funny-looking bottles. I personally refuse to pay a buck seventy-five for six ounces of plain water with fizz in it, regardless of what fancy foreign spring it shoots out of. Here's the Cheapo Goldberg Alternative, plain tap water. You can order it on the rocks, straight up, or with a twist. And best of all it's free, with NO calories.

ALCOHOL AND CALORIES:
THE PRICE YOU PAY

Alcoholic beverages are high in calories, but low in nutrients. People who want to lose weight, or maintain weight at a desirable level, should limit their intake of alcoholic beverages to their Cheating Day, to make room for foods with needed nutrients. The table below gives you an idea of how different alcoholic beverages compare in calories. Pay close attention to serving size when comparing items. A serving of beer is twelve fluid ounces—the size of the average bottle or can—while a serving of wine is only five fluid ounces—a little more than one-half cup. How big is *your* wine glass?

Compare the calories provided by alcohol and the calories provided by the energy-yielding nutrients in foods—fat, protein, and carbohydrates. You can see that alcohol provides more calories per gram than carbohydrates and protein, but less than fat.

ALCOHOLIC DRINKS	*APPROXIMATE CALORIES*
Beer	
Regular beer	12 fl. oz. = 150
Light beer	12 fl. oz. = 95
Liquor	(jigger = 1½ fl. oz.)
Gin, rum, vodka, and whiskey	
(86-proof)	jigger = 105
Vermouth, sweet	jigger = 70
Vermouth, dry	jigger = 55
Wine	
Sweet	5 fl. oz. = 200
Dry table, red	5 fl. oz. = 110
Dry table, white	5 fl. oz. = 115
Cordials and Liqueurs	jigger = 145

If you're making a mixed drink, you have to count the calories in the mixer, too.

CARBONATED DRINKS	*APPROXIMATE CALORIES*
Fruit-flavored	6 fl. oz. = 90
Root beer	6 fl. oz. = 80
Cola	6 fl. oz. = 80

Ginger ale	6 fl. oz. = 55
Quinine	6 fl. oz. = 60
Low-calorie soda (contains artificial sweeteners)	6 fl. oz. = 0–1
Club soda	6 fl. oz. = 0

FRUIT AND VEGETABLE JUICES (Unsweetened)	*APPROXIMATE CALORIES*
Pineapple	6 fl. oz. = 105
Orange	6 fl. oz. = 90
Grapefruit	6 fl. oz. = 75
Tomato	6 fl. oz. = 35

Remember: Fruit and vegetable juices provide you with vitamins and minerals in addition to calories. Alcohol and most carbonated beverages provide you with only calories.

CALORIES: ALCOHOL VERSUS FOODS

	Calories per Gram
Fat	9
Protein	4
Carbohydrates	4
Alcohol	7

DIET DOS

- Check with your doctor about Controlled Cheating, goal weight, exercise program, and cholesterol count.
- Eat a variety of food from all the food groups.
- Cut out all fats from your food.
- Exercise and exercise.
- Drink at least 6–8 glasses of *water* every day.
- Eat very slowly, putting your fork down after every bite. This is the hardest thing I've ever had to do, but it works.
- Eat breakfast like a king or queen, lunch like a prince or princess, and dinner like a pauper or pauperess.
- Be patient, dear Controlled Cheater, this is a lifetime program. Give it time to work.

YOU WILL LOSE WEIGHT, KEEP IT OFF, AND SMILE WHEN YOU GET ON THE SCALE. CONTROLLED CHEATING WORKS.

DIET DON'TS

- Don't fool yourself. On diet days, keep track of all the food you stuff into your mouth, including your fingers.
- Don't make excuses. If you goof and cheat on a diet day, it's okay. Be honest and get your tush back on Controlled Cheating.
- Don't drown your food with fats, oils, sugar, and salt on diet days.
- Don't eat unless you're hungry.
- Do not waste calories. Don't eat just to move your mouth. Talk a lot.
- Don't change your Cheating Day.

CONTROLLED CHEATING WORKS.

REFRIGERATOR RAPS

BY
1 LIVE JEW

Here's a poetic interlude to goose you through the fun-filled fourteen days.

DAY ONE

When Goldberg proposed this new diet
An overweight gal said, "I'll try it."
So she bought this book
And found what to cook—
"One potato—boil it—don't fry it!"

DAY TWO

Day Two is where you'll find me.
Not to eat you don't have to remind me,
'Cause I'm getting slimmer
Thinner and trimmer
And my behind is closer behind me.

DAY THREE

Now we're at Day the Third,
Where chewing can barely be heard.

Just keep on pickin'
That four ounces of chicken.
You're eating (just like) a bird.

DAY FOUR

The fourth day you get your great wish,
But only if it was for fish.
Don't sneer at your flounder,
He'd look a lot sounder
If he weren't so alone in that dish.

DAY FIVE

On the fifth day you see at a glance
It's easier to fit into your pants.
Soon your derrieres
Will be smaller than Cher's
And your waistlines won't look like Lou Grant's.

DAY SIX

You've come all the way to Day Six;
You don't need that old food fix.
Your shape's getting smaller,
You even feel taller,
Like you could play ball for the Knicks.

DAY SEVEN

Here we are at Day Seven.
That means we're halfway to heaven.
But forget about manna,
Just enjoy your banana—
Even Moses got only unleaven.

DAY EIGHT

It's all downhill at Day Eight.
You're looking and feeling just great.

No candy, no pies,
So who'll criticize
'Cause you're licking the crumbs off your plate?

DAY NINE

This day is like your ninth inning,
No wonder you're happy and grinning.
You've reached your dream,
You've made the "team,"
And what's more important, you're winning!

DAY TEN

You look so terrific, you "10,"
What a difference between now and then!
The ladies are able
To think you're Clark Gable;
To the men you're Sophia Loren.

DAY ELEVEN

This is the eleventh hour,
Of strength, you've become a tower.
You look sharp and lean
In your skin-tight jeans,
Thanks to less fats, less sugar, less flour!

DAY TWELVE

Twelve so becomes you, my dear,
We make such a wonderful pair.
From using less Crisco
You're ready to disco—
And folks think that I'm Fred Astaire.

DAY THIRTEEN

Thirteen was considered unlucky
'Til you came along, oh so plucky.

No ice cream breaks,
Or big two-pound steaks,
Or chicken, fried from Kentucky.

DAY FOURTEEN

The two longest weeks of your life
Have ended without any strife.
To the food war you stagger
Not with gun or with dagger,
Just a fork and a spoon and a knife!
Dig in!

WEIGHTY MATTERS

HOW TO FIGURE
YOUR GOAL WEIGHT

This one is all yours. The Old Cheater can suggest how and what to eat, what not to eat, and exercises to get you to your fighting weight. But only you and your doc can figure out your Goal Weight.

Goal Weight is something most overweight folks already know about themselves. If you're stuck, maybe you can peek at those insurance weight charts for a general guide.

I'll bet a Dairy Queen Peanut Buster Parfait that many of you know at what weight or size you felt most comfortable and looked your best. For women, it could be when they got out of school or got married or slipped into a string bikini. For guys, it could be when they buttoned their pants without sucking in half the air in the universe.

Whatever poundage you decide to lose, you must stick to your Goal Weight. The best news when you hit your goal weight is *You Get Another Cheating Day Every Week.* Wowee!

Plus you have a goal to shoot for. It's that beautiful light at the end of the diet tunnel. It's the summit of your

Controlled Cheating mountain. Put a flag in the whipped cream, take pictures, get on the "Today Show," and scream that you've conquered Mount Fatness.

Your Goal Weight? Whatever makes you healthy and happy.

ODE TO MY HEALTH-O-METER

When I die at the age of ninety-three, I want my faithful and trusty Health-O-Meter scale for my tombstone. If the cemetery won't allow ancient scales for headstones, then I'm going to have it buried with me in my plain pine box. They say you can't take it with you, but I'm going to prove them wrong. (Who are "they" anyway?)

No one knows what's on the other side. Maybe, just maybe, there will be a "Fat Heaven" where we can eat all we want and never get fat. What a heaven it would be, with cherry pies and apple tarts growing on trees and fettucini Alfredo sprouting from the ground. If this happens, then I'll still give my scale a proper place of honor, next to my hanging Pepsi plant.

Suppose, on the other hand, I have to diet for eternity. Then I'll surely need my scale. Any way I look at it, there's no way I'm leaving without it.

One reason why I'm not married is that I'm deeply in love with my scale. It's a real love/hate relationship, though. That sweetheart on the bathroom floor never lies. I've talked to it, cussed at it, and caressed it. The scale's my friend on thin days and I hate it on fat days, depending on where that big black needle stops.

The year I went from 325 to 190, I weighed myself when I got up, after I went to the bathroom, before I got dressed, when I came home from work, when I ate, after I ate, and before I went to bed. On weekends, in the middle of the afternoon, I'd strip down and weigh to see how things were going.

For thirty compulsive years, I twitched every morning about getting on that scale. My life was ruled by this hunk of metal and plastic grinning up at me from the floor.

Two years ago I finally screamed, "Enough! Out, out, damn scale!" (Sort of.)

Miracle of miracles, I now only weigh twice a week on the morning of my Cheating Days. That's enough.

MAGIC WITH THE SCALE
OR HOUDINI WITH THE HEALTH-O-METER

When it comes to con games and magic tricks with my scale, I make Paul Newman and Robert Redford in *The Sting* look like amateurs.

You probably have your own magic tricks hidden up your sleeves to make your scale read lighter. Alas, even for an old scale trickster like me, every magic act I try is only an illusion. If we're not getting our real weight, we're only kidding ourselves.

Heaven forbid that I corrupt you, but if you don't already know them, here are some of my old favorite hocus-pocus tricks.

1. SLEIGHT OF HAND: Also called Slight of Hand. Pick up your scale and move it to carpeting, which will make it register lighter than on a hard floor.
2. TIPPYTOE AND HEEL-ROCK BAMBOOZLE: Stand on your toes to make the dial go down. This is very hard on your toenails. Heel rock is the opposite. Rock back on your heels with caution. It could be dangerous due to the fact you may slide off and bounce into the bathtub. The problem with these tricks is that they don't work.
3. MAKING THE SCALE DISAPPEAR: This works very well if you wear glasses. It's a simple illusion. Do not wear your glasses when you weigh. Squinting at the dial will automatically let you read

a lower number. For those who don't wear glasses, think sad thoughts. Your eyes will tear and the scale will become a blur. Make up any weight you want.

4. THE SIDE BEND SNEAK: While standing on the scale, bend your body far to the right. When you look at the dial at this angle, the needle will appear farther to the left where the numbers are smaller.

5. TOWEL BAR ILLUSION: As you step on the scale, grab hold of the towel bar with one hand, put the other in the sink, and press down. This way you can weigh anything you want. The Towel Bar Illusion can also be performed with an assistant. Have another person stand next to you while you're on the scale. With your forearm, press down on the assistant's shoulder. You can also hold on to the wall or hang from the chandelier or shower curtain. If you use an assistant, make sure he or she has strong shoulders and is good-looking.

6. THE VANISHING ACT: This works very well. Throw the scale out, smash it to bits, or leave it at someone's doorstep. You can always say the scale was too old and you need to buy a new one. This trick was taught to me by my friend Judy, a professional scale magician. In the last three years she has smashed five scales beyond recognition. Judy now has an iron scale that is guaranteed indestructible. She recently retired from the profession.

All this trickery is top secret. Keep your magic scale illusions in your magic top hat along with your disappearing fat rabbit.

DO NOT MARCH TO A DIFFERENT SCALE

In the good old days, when I was checking my weight every twenty-five minutes, I'd daily drop by Marshall

Fields on State Street in Chicago and weigh on every scale on the rack to see if I weighed less on any of them. Finally the sales folks got tired of seeing me and inquired politely whether I'd like to purchase one. I explained I had already bought one there and this was a hobby for me—trying out new scales.

One courteous saleslady explained that the hobby department was on another floor, but I could have visiting privileges once a week to see my old pals.

I also weighed in at friends' houses and apartments, strange doctors' offices, or anywhere there was something with a platform and numbers that would tell me how much I weighed.

Weighing on every scale you see is dangerous. Just because you see a scale at someone's house, or in a department store, or even in the meat department of your supermarket doesn't mean you have to climb on. You weigh differently at different times during the day. You also have clothes on. And all scales weigh differently.

I know what you're doing, you little devil, you. You're looking for a friendly gauge that will give you a lower number so you can feel better and maybe cheat a little bit more. But no way. To play the scale like a professional, this is the only way to weigh:

Please weigh every day in the morning, on your own scale, without your clothes on.

THE CARE AND FEEDING OF THE SCALE
OR, TAKING CARE OF
YOUR FRIEND ON THE FLOOR

You might think that once you buy a scale, you just take it home, throw it on the floor, and you can forget about it. You think you'll never touch your scale again, except with your feet, when you climb on board every morning. Pals, scales don't work that way. They have hearts and souls just like you. You take care of your dog, cat, crocodile, and Model-A Ford, so why should your scale be any different?

I caress, fondle, and talk to my scale like the friend it is. Once a week, I bathe my yellow-covered baby with Mr. Clean (lemon scented) and wipe it dry with Bounty paper towels. I make doubly sure the plastic piece that covers the dial is crystal clear, so I can get an accurate picture of my weight.

I keep my scale in the bathroom. But any place is fine. The kitchen is good because it could give you a warning before you whip open the refrigerator door.

If I ever redecorate, I'm going to center my luxurious new living room around my scale. I'll use it as a piece of free-form sculpture, right next to my Sony twelve-inch color TV, across from my battered rolltop desk with its Smith-Corona typewriter.

My scale and I will shortly announce our engagement. You'll be invited to the wedding. We'll be registered at Safeway. Don't worry about sizes or colors.

WHY YOU SHOULD WEIGH EVERY DAY UNTIL YOU REACH YOUR GOAL WEIGHT

Yes, you should weigh every day until you reach your Goal Weight. After you reach your Goal Weight, you can weigh on the mornings of your Cheating Days.

Everyone in the diet, nutrition, and medical business, plus waitresses, bus drivers, and junk-bond dealers have their own theories about when, where, and how to weigh. What do they know? I know everything about weighing, and frankly, I've never seen anything about weighing yourself once a year. Probably the people who would tell you to weigh annually can't see the scale over their tummies.

I have my own pain-tested reasons why I hop on the scale every morning. For the better part of thirty years, I weighed every day because I liked good news. I wanted to boost my morale. I wanted to see how I was doing immediately. And eternal vigilance is the price of successful Controlled Cheating.

Also, I didn't want any big surprises. Every week or month was too long to wait. I wanted to see a number on that scale now.

Getting up, I made my bed (hooray for fitted sheets), shuffled into the bathroom naked (don't get excited), and got on the old Health-O-Meter. This is a sure waker-upper. All I have to do is hop on the scale and get a big surprise up or down and I wake up faster than if Michelle Pfeiffer were standing next to me.

Six or seven years ago, I tried weighing once a week. I could handle once a week on Saturday mornings, one of my Cheating Days. I'd been a successful skinny for twenty-five years. What could be bad? What could happen?

The first week was a breeze. I did my normal low-cal diet, hopped on the scale Saturday morning, and I was still at my original Goal Weight. This was easy and wonderful.

The second week I cheated on my two days. *But* on my Diet Days I started horsing around a little bit: another half a bagel here, a Fudge-sicle there. I said to myself, "Take it easy. You can take it off toward the end of the week and still come in under the wire at your original Goal Weight on Saturday morning."

Quit grinning! You guessed it. I danced up to the scale that Saturday morning and my farsighted eyes almost fell like marbles on the dial. I had slapped on four big ones over my Goal Weight.

I looked to see if anyone was standing on the scale with me. My palms became rivers of nervous perspiration. A deep rumble that started in my appendix careened up my quivering body, and as it escaped through my tortured teeth, it became a scream of terror.

That was it. No more weighing once a week. Everyday weighing was my one-way ticket to slimness.

Then a couple of years ago, I made a mighty resolution. The scale was not going to rule my life. So, I tried weighing *twice* a week, on the mornings of my Cheating Days, before breakfast, and before I shower. And bless my soul, it worked.

UPS AND DOWNS

Everybody loses weight at different rates. Some folks drop a lot at the beginning. Some don't lose for a while and then it clicks. Not everyone loses at the same rate. Everyone's staircase of weight loss is different, and some have landings.

Sometimes I get real cocky and smart-alecky about my body. I think I can play my body like Harry Connick Jr. can play the piano. No one watches what they eat and drink the way I do. If I eat certain diet foods, I'll lose so many pounds, I tell myself. Then I'm almost always shocked at how wrong I can be about forecasting my weight in the morning. So I stopped predicting. My body remains a mystery. Everyone loves a mystery.

My body also plateaus. No, don't get jealous if your body doesn't plateau. I just mean that there were times on my trip from 325 to 160 when I stayed at the same weight regardless of what I ate or didn't eat.

In 1959 there was a period when I got stuck at the same weight for about three weeks. I was eating the same amount of low-calorie food, but the dumb needle wasn't moving. I was going crazy. I didn't know what to do. What was going on? I got discouraged. Maybe God wanted me fat? No such luck. Finally I dropped five pounds in one day. Happily, I was off and running again.

Our weight fluctuates, especially when we're losing. Don't get discouraged if the dial does the Mamba. During the first weeks of dieting and Controlled Cheating, our bodies have to adjust to the new program.

There are physiological changes that arbitrarily happen that have nothing to do with how you're dieting and

Controlled Cheating. As long as you're following your low-calorie, balanced diet program, you'll be fine.

You are going to see fluctuations. The scale is a tough teacher. Don't let it throw you and Controlled Cheating out the window. There's no way you're going to see a weight loss every day. You have to accept that losses will come slowly.

Keep a close eye on your body and see how it operates. If it plateaus, relax and keep dieting. Eventually, you'll start skipping down those stairs again.

HIKING AND BIKING
WITH THE
JEWISH VIKING

Everybody up! Don't sit there. Time to start moving that gorgeous body. To lose a size, EXERCISE! Physical movement and a lifetime eating plan are the *only* way to lose weight and keep it off.

"Hiking" is the most important chapter in this book. You can diet, meditate, procrastinate, or fornicate, but nothing works like moving your tush.

FATS GOLDBERG SWEATS, OR, HOW A KID WHO WEIGHED 105 POUNDS IN THE THIRD GRADE, 240 POUNDS IN THE EIGHTH GRADE, AND 265 POUNDS IN HIGH SCHOOL, LEARNED HOW TO THROW A BASEBALL

SCHOOL DAYS, SCHOOL DAYS

Waddling out the back door of my house at the age of six or seven in Kansas City, I struggled over to the gym at Blessed Sacrament Catholic Church and School.

Those one hundred short yards were some of the most important steps of my fat young life. The Catholic school system started their kids in organized sports at an age when I was still trying to get enough coordination to tie my shoes.

Growing up (and sideways) in a predominantly Catholic neighborhood, my pals were the McGlynns, Rogerses, Kellys, Saladinos, Lopezes, Andersons, and Rineharts.

All of them were hot jocks at the age of ten. For me to hang around with them, I had to rouse myself and get out there and play, too. What I really wanted to do was sit on the curb and eat Fudge-sicles.

We played football, baseball, and basketball every free minute for years.

When I first started, I wasn't coordinated enough or strong enough to shoot the basketball and even hit the hoop. When we chose up teams, I was always picked next to last. The only reason why I wasn't picked last was because of Patty McGlynn, a girl who was two years younger and sixty pounds lighter. Now that I think about it, she *was* picked ahead of me quite a few times.

Finally, after several months, I was actually running and playing for hours. But I didn't lose any weight. No sir. When it got dark and we had to go home for dinner, I hopped into Goldberg's Market like a famished, crazed kangaroo.

We played regardless of snow, rain, or heat straight through grade school, high school, and halfway through college.

Thanks to the other guys, the gym, and the tiny baseball field between the church and school, I developed coordination and strength. Without them, I probably couldn't even walk down the street without tripping.

GOLDBERG'S MARKET

What also helped my coordination and strength was delivering groceries for Goldberg's Market, "Fancy Groceries and Meats, Free Delivery." (I was the free delivery.)

Sara and Art Goldberg had me on one of those Schwinn Cycle Trucks. You know, the bicycle with the big basket and small wheel on the front. I was hauling "Fancy Groceries and Meats" all over the hilly place. But I didn't lose weight riding that bike, either. Every time I came panting back from a delivery, it was a Mason's Root Beer and a Dolly Madison Banana Flip.

BOY SCOUTS AND SWIMMING

All right, so I'm not an Eagle Scout. But I am a Life Scout. I didn't get my Eagle Scout Badge because I was afraid of deep water and couldn't get Swimming and Life Saving merit badges.

Given the large surface area of my spongy body, though, I was a world champion floater. I sure did love the water and was a great shallow-water swimmer. I knew all the life-saving strokes and carries. Still, if I couldn't put my foot down and touch bottom, sheer panic would overcome my quivering form.

I'm fifty-seven years old and still get teased about not being an Eagle Scout. I even called the Boy Scouts of America a couple of months ago to see if I could get my Eagle. They said I was a little too old: the maximum age is eighteen.

GOLF AND CADDYING

Golf is one of my all-time favorite sports. I know people call it "barnyard pool" or "a pleasant little walk in the country." I was never very good. Still, schlepping around a beautiful golf course is wonderful.

I caddied for three years as a kid at Mission Hills Country Club in Kansas City. Used to make good bucks, too. I carried mostly "doubles"; one bag on each shoulder plus one pint of ice cream in each hand. With my weight, plus the weight of the golf bags, I developed muscles in my legs like a draft horse.

YOUR FIRST EXERCISE: Walk to the telephone. Curl up the receiver to your ear. Walk your fingers over the buttons and call your doctor. Check before you do anything more strenuous than picking your teeth.

TAKE A WALK

A LOVE LETTER

My dearest darling Walking:

We first met in 1959 in Chicago, where I was a dieting fat guy who thought a long walk was from my beige plastic chair to the refrigerator.

Then you tenderly took my hand and showed me Michigan Avenue, the Loop, Rush Street, Old Town, and, in the summer, the Oak Street Beach with the sand rushing between my toes and me staring at rows of beautiful women in bikinis. What an exciting world you opened to me.

In 1965, inflamed with love, you and I ran away to New York. Little did I know at the time, my sweet, that New York is one of the world's greatest walking experiences.

How can I forget, even after all these lovely, blissful thirty-two years with you, that there is a new street spectacular every ten feet; that walking boredom is unknown; that those concrete corridors beg to be trod by our cute Nike-shod feet; that our four- or five-mile daily walk has kept me lean; that, without you, my love, my pants would still have a forty-eight-inch waist.

What I admire about you is that you, Walking, are natural, no additives. Yes, humans were built to walk because we stand erect. Baby, we walk all the time.

You probably don't realize this about yourself, silly, but walking is the best all-around exercise there is.

You love everyone; with no age barriers, old, young, and in-between can walk. And we can walk with you all our romantic lives. You even welcome folks with some disabilities who can benefit from your love.

Precious Walking, most anyone can do it. You demand no special training, clothes, or equipment, only comfortable walking shoes. I wear running shoes to move more quickly beside you. The weather doesn't stop us either. What you are is a cheap passionate date, every man's dream.

But our most fun date is when we meet friendly women, neighbors, and nice dogs—planning our Controlled Cheating Day, learning about our neighborhood, and making new pals and lovers everywhere.

You're so adaptable and giving, sweetheart. We can work you into any of our strange life-styles. We can walk to work, walk to lunch, walk after dinner, walk to the store. Walk, walk, walk, you darling little fool.

Ha, angel, you do have your little regulations, don't you? We must walk briskly at the rate of three miles an hour for thirty minutes a day. And we should walk with a steady rhythm, breathing deeply and swinging our arms. You always remind us that when we get tired we should sit down and rest before going on.

Plus, light of my life, we must be consistent and walk every day, maybe taking the whole family along or walking with a friend or friends.

Walking, you're so good for us physically and mentally. We sleep better and walking improves circulation, blood to the heart, and helps reduce blood pressure. You also help us build muscle strength. Nervous? Tense? Troubled? Take a walk and clear the brain.

Sweet patootie, you're so wonderful for folks who are flabby, out of shape, or nonathletic. You won't hurt us like other exercises that are so strenuous.

My favorite times with you, devoted one, are when we

eat and walk at the same time. Funny me. I know it burns up calories.

After eating is also one of my favorite times with you. Time for using up more of those ugly little calories.

Buttercup, you probably don't know about this yourself, but if a 150-pound person walks for an hour, four days a week, at three miles an hour, he will lose about twelve pounds a year—if he eats the same amount of food as he did before walking. If he eats less, then he'll lose even more weight.

Honey bunch, snookums, I must tear myself away from you now.

We shall meet again when I tie on my Nikes.

I miss you already, heart of hearts.

You will always be my perfect "10" in the exercise department.

XOXOXOXOXOXOXOXOXOXOXOX

Fats

The world is walking a path to your door.

HUFFIN' AND PUFFIN' 'TIL YOU'RE DOWN TO NUTHIN'

- YOU MUST EXERCISE TO BE A CONTROLLED CHEATER.
- You have to burn the calories you ate on your Cheating Day.
- You'll feel terrific with the energy of a space shot.
- Exercise does wonders for your dear heart and circulation.
- Exercise is the Comet Cleanser of the mind. No more fuzz, lint, crazy notions, or anything else clogging your mind.
- Great for muscle toning and tension easing.
- You'll fall asleep quicker and sleep better.
- You can walk anywhere or any place.

- Walk alone or with a pal. It's very social. Especially with the opposite sex.
- A 160-pound person walking four miles an hour burns 375 calories and keeps on burning them for another 12 hours. Starting at one or two years old, you've been walking all your life. You're already a professional.
- Hungry? Take a walk.
- Gently stretch before you walk.
- Regular walking burns calories, reduces risk of heart disease, lowers blood pressure and bone loss, and you can eat more. Yeah.
- Get off the bus or subway two or three stops before your destination and walk.
- Make walking exciting. Crank up your imagination.
- A recent study shows you can extend your life by two years if you burn just two thousand calories a week in all physical activity, which is about three hours of brisk walking plus other physical stuff like raking the leaves, painting the garage, cleaning out the basement, or flying a kite.
- You can meet other folks, fall in like, listen to the birdies, stare at the trees, and sweat.
- Regardless of how much you tip the scales at, or how out of shape you are, you can still walk and do it the rest of your life.
- Indoor walking? Malls are best. There are about three thousand malls in the USA just waiting for you. Malls are safe, quiet, no big dogs or hysterical cats, the air is good, no cars or their exhaust fumes, no bugs, and maybe you can meet a pal.
- Call any of the Y's about the availability of a track or treadmill.
- "Talk Test": You should be able to carry on a conversation while schlepping. If you get breathless, you're going too fast.

- Walking is a hunger killer.
- One foot is always on the ground; that's why walking is almost injury free. Unless you get in a fight with your walking friend.
- Exercise makes Controlled Cheating work.
- You'll eat smarter because you're working your body into fine shape.
- Each mile you walk burns one hundred calories.
- Walking helps you to stop smoking. You need good lungs.
- Old age will never catch you.
- Over four hundred thousand folks walk to work in the USA.
- Walking is cheap. You only need a good pair of walking shoes.
- Remember it takes 3500 calories to put on a pound of fat. And you have to use 3500 calories to take it off—START WALKING!
- Bring the family along. Have a party. No arguing allowed.
- Drink plenty of water before and after you walk.

TO START YOUR WALKING PROGRAM

1. Move your rear out of the recliner.
2. Walk at a comfortable speed.
3. Walk every other day.
4. Build your walking up to thirty minutes, then to forty-five minutes or more, five times a week.
5. Aim for a fifteen-minute mile pace.
6. YOU WILL NOT KEEP THE WEIGHT PERMANENTLY OFF IF YOU DO NOT KEEP WALKING.

Walking is the most fun of any aerobic exercise.
You'll laugh with every step.
Your upper body also needs a workout. Bend your

arms at ninety degrees and move them smartly back and forth like a pendulum. Working your arms and legs makes walking a total-body aerobic exercise.

Park your dumb car at the farthest corner of the mall parking lot and walk.

Take the stairs. Forget the elevator or escalator. Walking up stairs burns four calories every ten steps.

WALKING WHILE TRAVELING

1. Walk, don't take taxis.
2. Walk up and down the hotel halls.
3. Stay in hotels with gyms and use their treadmills.
4. Walk in airports. You could even get there an hour earlier.

The fitness motto that flashes on every corner is: WALK! Don't run.

Our bodies are better suited to walking than to sitting, standing, or running.

Work walking into your daily routine.

MARATHONING

At the age of fifty-three, I wanted to see if I could walk a marathon. There's an organization in New York, now worldwide, called the Achilles Track Club. The runners are disabled and they need volunteers to walk with them in the New York City Marathon. I now have walked four marathons with the Achilles Track Club. This is probably the single best activity in my life. What's funny is that I need them more than they need me.

HUGGIN' AND KISSIN'

Hugging and kissing are great exercise mentally and physically for any and all occasions. The three best things in the world are hugging and kissing, pizza, and air conditioning—not necessarily in that order.

Hugging and kissing is the number one, best, alltime cure for the diet blues. As Dr. Theodore Rubin, the famous formerly fat psychiatrist, says, "Next time you're hungry, reach for your mate instead of your plate."

What else can I say about huggin' and kissin' that you haven't already thought of, and probably practice better than I do? Only the following:

This is a public service announcement that will eliminate confusion and be of great help in using sex to lose pounds. Here are the actual calories used per hour during sex. Really, this no joke.

CALORIES USED PER HOUR DURING SEX*

Weight	110 lbs.	150 lbs.	200 lbs.
	Calories used	Calories used	Calories used
Foreplay	80	100	115
Intercourse			
a. Aggressor	235	300	350
b. Submissor	105	135	155

*From: *The Exerciser's Handbook* by Charles Kuntzleman, Ph.D., National YMCA Consultant, David McKay Company, Inc., Publishers; Copyright 1978.

These calories refer to calories used per hour. If the sex act lasts fifteen minutes, simply divide by four; twenty minutes by three; thirty minutes by two; and so on.

PERSONAL OBSERVATIONS
FROM FATS GOLDBERG

This chart fails to take into consideration wild foreplay in a hot room on an August afternoon in The Acme Motel on Route 66 in Braceville, Illinois. I personally have lost three to five pounds in such activity, besides curling my hair and clearing my skin.

I love this kind of chart. You will, too. You can do all sorts of calculations on the best exercise or combination to counteract conspicuous calorie consumption.

This little beauty shows you how many minutes of physical activity it takes to burn up different high-calorie goodies.

BIG TIME CHART #1
FOR CALORIES USED IN VARIOUS FORMS
OF PHYSICAL MESSING AROUND

MINUTES OF EXERCISE

FOOD	Calories	Jogging	Swimming	Bicycling	Walking	Lying Down
Hamburger	350	18	31	43	67	269
Doughnut	150	8	13	18	29	116
Beer, 1 glass	115	6	10	14	22	88
Pie, apple, 1/6	375	19	34	46	73	290
Strawberry shortcake	400	21	36	49	77	308
Chicken, TV dinner	540	28	48	66	104	417
Ice Cream Soda	255	13	23	31	49	196

BIG TIME CHART #2 FOR CALORIES USED
BY A 150-POUND PERSON IN ALL SORTS OF
PHYSICAL ACTIVITY PER HOUR

Rest and Light Activity	Calories
Lying down or sleeping	80
Sitting	100
Driving an automobile	120
Standing	140
Domestic work	180

Moderate Activity

Bicycling (5½ mph)	210
Walking (2½ mph)	210

Moderate Activity (con't.)	Calories
Gardening	220
Canoeing	230
Golf	250
Lawn mowing (power mower)	250
Lawn mowing (hand mower)	270
Bowling	270
Fencing	300
Rowboating (2½ mph)	300
Swimming (¼ mph)	300
Walking (3¾ mph)	300
Badminton	350
Horseback riding (trotting)	350
Square dancing	350
Volleyball	350
Roller skating	350

Vigorous Activity	
Table tennis	360
Ditch digging (hand shovel)	400
Ice skating (10 mph)	400
Wood chopping or sawing	400
Tennis	420
Water skiing	480
Hill climbing (100 ft. per hour)	490
Skiing (10 mph)	600
Squash and handball	600
Cycling (13 mph)	660
Scull rowing (race)	840
Running (10 mph)	900

THE VERY BEST EXERCISE IN THE WORLD IS TO PUSH YOURSELF AWAY FROM THE TABLE.

CHEATIN' EATIN'

Congrats, wowee, zap, zoweee, you've made it to your first Controlled Cheating Day. In all your natural (no additives), long, healthy life, you will never have to diet for longer than six days without cheating.

Turn around real quick and look back on the last fourteen days. You can do this a lot easier now because you've even lost pounds and inches off your shoulders. Those days weren't too tough for a low-cal cookie like you, were they? Your diet gave you plenty to eat. It was balanced, and all those nourishing nutrients energized you enough to roof the house with one-inch squares, mow the lawn with a pair of scissors, and play three sets of tennis with a racquet with no strings, all on Saturday morning before eleven-thirty.

With all those nifty food choices in the eating plan, you can move around and up and down the diet and slay Boredom, that old diet dragon, with the Golden Sword of Variety. Even when your Controlled Cheating Day is over, you can return to your diet without a whimper or a tear.

YOUR CHEATING DAY IS AS IMPORTANT AS THE DIET

CONTROLLED CHEATING IS HEALTHY

The biggest, largest, grandest reason I know Controlled Cheating is healthy is that I'm sitting here on a rainy Saturday afternoon staring at my humming Smith-Corona and pounding away with my ten bony fingers.

When I was fat, the doctors said I'd be lucky to reach thirty. I'm now fifty-seven years old, in the best shape of my life, except for an occasional stretch mark, and I never get sick. Once in a while I do get a sore throat—but that's from keeping my head too long in ice cream freezers.

The hypochondria got so bad by the time I was in college that a friend had to rip the Medicine section out of *Time* magazine before I could read it. As soon as I started losing weight, I lost the hypochondria. Now I'm thin and cured.

But back to the doctors. They all said the same thing: "Goldberg, you sure do like your groceries. You've got to lose weight. Instead of a Tootsie Roll, pick up an apple." They didn't know who they were talking to. I thought the only apples in the world were grown in Dutch apple pie, with a sugary, crunchy top and raisins and heavy cinnamon.

Then these same M.D.s would hand me the usual mimeographed sheet with the usual diet. The diet was always the same. Breakfast: half a grapefruit, one soft-boiled egg, one piece of dry whole wheat toast, a glass of skim milk, and coffee or tea with no sugar or cream. Lunch and dinner were even more terrible. I was supposed to stay on *that* the rest of my life?

But I always started the following morning with mighty resolve. By 8:35 A.M. I had both hands rammed in a sack of nutty Danishes. That blew that diet for another seven months.

Almost every medical, nutritional, and diet expert I've talked to, read about, seen, or heard gives the same advice to folks who want to lose weight and keep it off: Don't eliminate any food from your diet; rather, cut down the quantities you eat. That's wise advice, *if* you can control yourself twenty-four hours a day, seven days a week, twelve months of every year of your whole life. I can't.

What they don't understand is how true fat people eat. There's not a chubby alive who can stop eating a hunk of fresh banana cake with chocolate ice cream after four bites. If they put a tiny sliver on the plate with a thimble of ice cream, it *will not* satisfy a real fatty. If a plumperoo could eat that way, he wouldn't be fat in the first place.

No one ever sat down and figured out how fat people eat. I had to think it through because I was going nowhere with every other diet plan. If I didn't do something, I knew in my soul that I would keep blowing up until I was the size of the Goodyear Blimp and explode in a couple of years.

I did take their health advice, but I switched it all around. I knew I had to diet, but I just couldn't give up my favorite foods for the rest of my life. So, I kept all the good stuff confined to one day a week for starters. Then I could be a free man in the morning when the diet began, because I knew I'd get to see my food friends soon.

Bang. Controlled Cheating leapt in on little pig's feet. I saved all my Controlled Cheating calories for one outstanding day a week where I could eat everything and anything my heart desired.

At that moment, my 325-pound body wobbled with joy at the coming good health and sighed deeply with relief at the prospect of the 175-pound licorice anvil I was going to lift off its back. Everyone was happy.

CONTROLLED CHEATING FLIPS YOUR LID, OR, TAKE OFF YOUR DIETER'S DERBY

You're wearing an invisible, tight-fitting hat. You don't see it, but boy, you can feel it. I call it the Dieter's Derby, and it's automatically crammed on anyone who ever thought about pouring a fistful of cashews into his mouth. The Dieter's Derby comes only in black—with no feather. There are no pinks, chartreuses, or mauves. The Derby is not something you wear to the Easter Parade.

The mind-numbing tightness comes from always having to think about what you're going to eat and how many calories it has. Will the needle shoot up when you jump on the scale tomorrow morning? Do you really want that hot dog with sauerkraut? Sam or Samantha said you were getting a little heavy: shoot, are you going to eat that bag of chocolate chip cookies or not? Decisions, decisions, decisions.

See, there's this constant tension from always having to think about dieting and losing weight, and making decisions on what and how much you're going to eat. That ugly-as-mud Dieter's Derby was one of my biggest problems. All the other diets I'd tried were for seven horrible days and nights a week, every week for endless weeks. My head was like a giant volcano ready to explode with a strawberry milk shake pouring down my slopes. No relief was in sight.

Finally I discovered Controlled Cheating, and the Dieter's Derby disappeared. Yes, just like at graduating ceremonies, you can throw your Dieter's Derby in the air and it evaporates on your Controlled Cheating Days. With Controlled Cheating Days, all the tautness, pressure, and tightness are gone.

As Humphrey Yogurt once said, "Hat's off to you, kid."

CONTROLLED CHEATING IS GUILT-FREE
The Skinny World vs.
Tammy and Teddy Thunder Thighs

JUDGE CRACKER: Jury, have you reached a verdict?

JURY: Yes, Your Honor, we have. We find the defendants guilty on all charges:

1. Eating a Wonder bread and Miracle Whip salami sandwich and washing it down with an apple fritter while supposedly on a diet.

2. Sneaking three tablespoons of turkey dressing at 2:30 A.M. on Thanksgiving morning, 1965.

3. Lifting four and a half french fries from their daughter Tara's tray at McDonald's.

4. Scraping the top off of three slices of sausage and pepperoni pizza while screaming, "I never eat the crust; it's so fattening." Then four minutes later starting to nibble until all three crusts were gone.

JUDGE CRACKER: The jury has found you guilty on all counts. Do you have anything to say in your defense before I pass sentence?

T & T: Yes, Your Honor. Who squealed?

JUDGE CRACKER: That's it? I should sentence both of you to a life term of gooey guilt, to be served in the Fat Slammer of Dumb Diets. However, being merciful, I will parole both of you to Controlled Cheating. Your parole officer is to be General Goldberg.

T & T: Oh, thank you, thank you. We look forward to it. Huzzah, huzzah for Judge Cracker.

NOT GUILTY

Controlled Cheating *will* take all the guilt from Cheating Eating because it is *planned*. You know what you're going to do seven days a week. Controlled Cheating takes the tremendous weight of gooey guilt off your mind and stomach. Even without losing a pound the first day of your diet, you'll feel tons lighter.

For the first twenty-five years of my life, I carried around enough guilt about eating to make the gang in Sing Sing look as innocent as "The Cosby Show." Snatching handfuls of Hydrox cookies from Goldberg's Market, running to the back room, and stuffing them down: guilty. Stealing money from my thrifty, skinny sister Jocelyn to buy chocolate ice cream sodas: guilty. Grabbing meatloaf from friends' plates in high school when they left to get a glass of water: guilty. Riffling the drawers of fraternity brothers at 2:00 A.M., when they'd gotten a goody package from home: guilty. Making homesick campers cry at Boy Scout Camp in Osceola, Missouri, so they couldn't eat and I could clean their plates: guilty.

But hey, don't put the cuffs on me yet—I've repented. I used to feel guilty, but no more. Why? Because guilt from eating comes from uncontrollable eating when you aren't supposed to. With Controlled Cheating, you know what you're doing every minute of every day, especially on your Cheating Day when you've planned all of the goodies you're going to eat.

What a relief!

YOU AIN'T SUPPOSED TO MESS WITH YOUR CONTROLLED CHEATIN' DAY, NO HOW

Once you've made the rock-hard choice of what Cheating Day you want, *that day cannot change*. Not for now, anyway. I want you to wait until you're firmly in the Controlled Cheating groove before we talk about that. Let me give you the reasons.

Suppose you've picked Saturday for your Controlled Cheating Day. Every Saturday you wake up happy as a hot dog in yellow mustard. Your Controlled Cheating program is doing fine. You're losing weight and feeling great. Then comes an invitation for a Sunday outdoor barbecue of sirloin steaks, homemade potato salad, baked beans with brown sugar, fresh-baked bread, tart cherry pie, and three barrels of cold soda pop.

STOP! Wait a minute. You cannot change your Cheating Eating Day.

I know you because I'm just like you. When you start switching Controlled Cheating Days for every dogfight and worm wrestle, you're headed for big Trouble with a capital T.

You'll not only cheat on that special Cheating Day, you'll cheat again on your regular Cheating Day.

Right now you're in a happy groove. Don't mess around with success. Otherwise you'll be back, ramming it in every day with both fists like you did before. Us fatties are sneaky.

The reason why Controlled Cheating works 100 percent of the time is that you can go through the toughest, hungriest days of your life because you can look forward to that wonderful Cheating Eating Day. It's special. Keep it that way. Savor it and you will not feel deprived, self-pitying, hurt, or martyred, because you've got that one hot fudge sundae day on the horizon.

I know it's a rigid life now, but it's a happy, thin life, and eventually you'll have more flexibility—I promise.

FATS GOLDBERG'S HIT LIST

Your Cheating Day is here. All the preliminary matches are over and it's time to rip the gloves off for the main event. The winner and still champion is: You and Controlled Cheating. "Happy Day is Here Again." You can eat *anything* and *everything* and *as much as you want.* All the Diet Derbies, guilts, and hungers are forgotten for today. Your teeth are ready for action.

On the mornings of my Controlled Cheating Days, I wake up with the birds and sing like a nasal lark. As I lay in bed staring up at my white cottage cheese ceiling, joy shoots through my body and I leap ecstatically straight up.

Skip ahead. This is my Hit List. You can probably add a few hundred of your own. I think I slapped on a couple of pounds just reading these names. Cheating Eating has been my life for nigh on to thirty-two years. In all that time, there's one piece of wisdom I've learned:

MAKE YOUR CONTROLLED CHEATING DAY SPECIAL

When I talk about making your Cheating Day special, I'm telling you to plan your menu in advance. But it's okay to deviate. Suppose you're strolling by a store that day and you get a crazy craving for macadamia nut brittle. Great. Add it on.

Planning ahead means cheating with the foods you truly, deeply love. It's really very romantic. Don't waste calories on any old food because it's there. Eat your heart's desire to your heart's content, but do it with love. Enjoy, savor, and eat your goodies slowly.

At the end of the big day, as you're slumped in the recliner full and happy, you'll be able to look back over the day with satisfaction and affection. You won't think back and moan, my God, why did I eat that white gummy roll with margarine. You should not use up valuable calories and space in the stomach department with foods that you are only lukewarm about. Be red hot about everything you gorge on.

Again, though, this is *your* fun day. You can eat your way through the Dolly Madison cake plant or you can have five fettucinis in forty minutes, or you can walk around your favorite mall going from Dairy Queen to Taco Bell to Arthur Bryant's Barbecue to Kentucky Fried Chicken.

GREASE, DOUGH, AND SUGAR

The greatest foods in all the world, the ones that are going to enrich your life, fall mainly, as I've said, into one or more of three magnificent categories: grease, dough, and sugar.

Some, which I consider superfoods, like glazed doughnuts and cheeseburgers loaded with mustard, fit into all three categories because of the scrumptious nature of their ingredients.

Unlike on your Diet Days, when you have to consider the basic food groups we're supposed to eat from for a balanced diet, on your Cheating Day you can hop, skip, and jump back and forth from the groups without a single thought about nutrition to ruin your day.

I ate only from grease, dough, and sugar to lift me to my stupendous 325 big ones. But remember that every day of my first twenty-five years was a Cheating Day—and uncontrolled at that.

Now we're reversing the situation. We're using those three groups not to make you fat, but, in a careful controlled way, to help you lose weight and keep it off. You can believe the Controlled Cheating diet allows you to enjoy these foods on your special day.

These lists are only a sampling from a small group of my all-time favorites. Feel free to cheat with any favorite of yours that I've overlooked. If you have any old family recipes laying around, or regional favorites of dynamite cheating foods, please write immediately with full instructions so I can expand my own cheating horizons.

*GREASED LIGHTNING: A FAST FOOD FANTASY**

Breakfast Meals	Calories
Egg McMuffin, orange juice (McDonald's)	407
English muffins w/2 butters, low-fat milk (McDonald's)	493
Hotcakes w/syrup/butter, orange juice (Carl's Jr.)	560
Scrambled egg, toast w/marg., coffee w/cream/sugar (Wendy's)	494
Scrambled eggs, bacon, coffee w/cream/sugar (Wendy's)	354
Ham & Swiss croissant, milk, orange juice (Arby's)	560
Cheese omelette, milk (Carl's Jr.)	440
Ham & egg biscuit, orange juice, coffee (Hardee's)	541
Crescent sandwich/sausage, coffee w/cream/sugar (Roy Rogers)	503
Pancake breakfast w/syrup, bacon, milk (Jack-in-the-Box)	767
Steak & egg biscuit, hash rounds, coffee w/2 sugars (Hardee's)	775

Lunch, Dinner Meals

Salad bar (peas, broccoli, cauliflower, romaine, reduced calorie dressing), orange juice (Wendy's)	203
Lightly breaded chicken, plain baked potato, water (D'Lites)	400
Fish fillet sandwich, plain baked potato, coffee (D'Lites)	510
Stuffed potato, chicken a la king, milk (Wendy's)	500
Roast beef (large), potato w/marg., water (Roy Rogers)	634
Sirloin steak dinner, coffee (Jack-in-the-Box)	699
Roast beef sandwich, fries, Coke (Roy Rogers)	730
Hamburger, Coke, apple pie (McDonald's)	652
King roast beef, plain potato, vanilla shake (Arby's)	1052
Catfish (3 pcs.), hush puppies (3 pcs.), fries, Coke (Church's)	835
Original white special dinner, Coke (Kentucky Fried Chicken)	748
Chicken McNuggets, fries, vanilla shake (McDonald's)	886
Fillet-O-Fish, fries, Coke (McDonald's)	796
Chicken strips dinner, vanilla shake (Jack-in-the-Box)	1009
Big Deluxe, fries, Coke (Hardee's)	929
Chicken breast sandwich, plain potato, vanilla shake (Arby's)	1177
Original combination special dinner, Coke (Kentucky Fried Chicken)	805
Quarter Pounder/cheese, fries, Coke (McDonald's)	888
Extra crispy white special dinner, Coke (Kentucky Fried Chicken)	899

Big Mac, fries, Coke (McDonald's)	927
Fish sandwich platter, carbonated drink (Long John Silver's)	955
Cheeseburger, fries, Coke (Roy Rogers)	869
Extra crispy dark special dinner, Coke (Kentucky Fried Chicken)	909
Hamburger, fries, vanilla shake, apple pie (Burger King)	1190
Whopper, onion rings, medium Pepsi (Burger King)	1041
Double cheeseburger, fries, Frosty, cola (Wendy's)	1420
Fish & More, Coke (Long John Silver's)	1096
Triple cheeseburger, fries, cola (Wendy's)	1430
Pepperoni pizza (3 slices), Coke (Pizza Hut)	710

*Reprinted from "Fast Food Guide," which is available from the Center for Science in the Public Interest, 1875 Connecticut Avenue, N.W. #300, Washington, D.C. 20009, for $4.95, copyright 1986.

CLASSIC GOLDBERG

Breakfast	Calories
Aunt Jemima buttermilk pancakes (3 cakes)	300
Two tablespoons butter	200
Three tablespoons Log Cabin Syrup	150
Midmorning Snack	
M&M Peanut candy, small bag	300
Lunch	
Pastrami Sandwich, 8 oz. on two slices rye bread w/ mustard	510
Small bag of potato chips	160
Pepsi Cola	150
Midafternoon Snack	
Popcorn, butter and salt added, 6 cups	240
Pepsi Cola	150
Dinner	
One-half fried chicken	950
Mashed potatoes	250
Biscuits & butter	250
Coca-Cola	150
Apple pie a la mode	400
Bedtime Snack	
Frozen Snickers Ice Cream Bar	300
Total Calories	4070

ALL-AMERICAN DAY
Star-Spangled Eating

Breakfast	Calories
2 large fried eggs	
3 slices fried bacon	
2 biscuits	
1 tablespoon butter	
1 glass of milk	785
Midmorning Snack	
Hydrox cookies, 6 cookies	300
Lunch	
McDonald's Big Mac	560
French fries	220
Chocolate shake	380
Midafternoon Snack	
Frozen Milky Way	270
Dinner	
1 pound sirloin steak	1200
1 baked potato with sour cream	220
Coca-Cola	150
Homemade apple pie, ⅙ of 9-inch pie with	
¼ pint vanilla ice cream	550
Bedtime Snack	
M&M peanut candy, small bag	300
Total Calories	4935

JUST DESSERTS
The Sweetest Day of Your Life

Breakfast	Calories
3 glazed doughnuts	450
Chocolate milk	200
Midmorning Snack	
Chocolate-chip cookies, 4	200
Lunch	
Banana cream pie, ⅓ of 9-inch pie, homemade	550
Lemonade	150
Midafternoon Snack	
Chocolate eclair, custard filled	325

Dinner

Sara Lee frozen cream cheesecake, 1 whole cake	850

Bedtime Snack

Hostess Twinkies, 2	320
Milk shake, any flavor	310

Optional

24 glasses of ice water	000
Total Calories	3355

SUPERMARKET SCHLEP
Instant Eats

Breakfast	**Calories**
Drake coffee cake	220
Fresh orange juice, 2 cups	225
Midmorning Snack	
Fig Newtons, 5 cookies	300
Lunch	
2 salami sandwiches (4 slices of rye bread, 10 slices of salami, plenty of hot mustard)	650
Pepsi Cola	150
Midafternoon Snack	
Snicker's candy bar	275
Dinner	
Chicken salad, ½ lb., 2 bagels	800
Dorito's tortilla chips	180
Coca-Cola	150
Bedtime Snack	
Hagen Daz Ice Cream, rum raisin, 1 big dip	275
Total Calories	3225

CHECKLIST FOR CHEATING ONCE A WEEK

- Cheat
- Plan your Cheating Day
- Exercise
- Drink Water
- Eat only when hungry. You'll enjoy it more.

- Never skip a Cheating Day.
- Never move your Cheating Day.
- Never put restrictions on your Cheating Day.
- Eat slowly—enjoy every bite. If the food doesn't taste good, don't eat it!
- Do not get up at 12:01 in the morning of your Cheating Day and start stuffing yourself. That is *uncontrollable cheating*. Leap out of bed at your normal time.

The philosophy of the Cheating Day is vital to the success of Controlled Cheating. That freedom and guilt-free feeling on a Cheating Day is almost sweeter than the most delicious, fattening food you will enjoy when you cheat. We all love to eat. Now we get to enjoy it. We've earned it.

A good Cheating Day can make or break the rest of the week. If the Cheating Day wasn't terrific—or you tried to put restrictions on the goodies—you'll feel like a brussels sprout.

Think about the entire day of guilt-free eating when you grab something you shouldn't on a diet. Is it worth giving all that up—the pure glory of your Cheating Day? Then go exercise.

Cheating without guilt is a learned freedom. You'll learn to love it.

Be happy . . . you're losing weight . . . *and keep cheating.*

THE DAY AFTER YOUR CHEATING DAY YOU MUST RETURN TO YOUR DIET

Welcome back. Had a good time? You don't want to come back? You want to keep cheating? Sure, I can understand that. Life was so terrific yesterday. You ate everything you wanted. You felt full and good. Wining, dining, running, and funning around. All those screaming fat cells finally quieted down for a while.

These next twenty-four hours are so important that I'm taking a whole chapter to bring your barbecued balloon back to earth. This is the most crucial, critical, twitchy day in your diet life. Hold on. I don't want to lose you. We both need all the company and help we can get.

Now you're back down to earth. Yesterday went so fast. All your taste buds got into a tizzy with all that action. Everything tasted so good. Many foods your taster had almost forgotten. But didn't those Cheating Eating foods taste ten times better? You hadn't eaten any of those goodies for two weeks. Didn't that make your Controlled Cheating Day even more fun? Absence makes the tummy grow fonder.

91

USE YOUR POWER.

Now don't roll over and bury your face in the pillow and start sobbing and beating your little fists against the injustice of it all.

Forget it. You've got to exercise your tough discipline and exorcise your food demons. After a Cheating Eating Day, you feel caught in a velvet vise. They've got you "in between the devil's food cake and the deep dish blueberry pie."

I know those food demons are prancing back and forth on your down-filled comforter and running up and down the walls and ceiling grinning with their lime-flavored Life Saver teeth. Some of your tempting, delicious pals are beckoning, taunting, and whispering in your ear: "Come with us for another day. Remember those buttery hash brown potatoes? So what if you can't button your pants, you sweat all the time, and your bowling score should be as high as your blood pressure. We've been friends for years. We need you, buddy, more than one day a week. What do ya say, Plumperoo?"

Shut your eyes and scream, "Out, out, damn demons. Be gone. I want no further truck with you for six full days. I shall remember you often, all of you, for we shall meet again in six short days. Who can forget the wonderful times we had yesterday? I'm already planning which ones of you I'm going to be seeing next week on that GREAT COME-AND-GET-IT DAY."

YOUR SLIMMER SLAMMER

This is the day after your Controlled Cheating Day and you must sentence yourself to go back to the Slimmer Slammer.

This Slimmer Slammer is a maximum-security jail for hardened fatties, located on an island paradise in your mind (next to the Statue of Liberty, that beautiful lady who represents your Cheating Day). It's a Big House from which you parole yourself once a week. You've sentenced yourself there because you're the warden, guard, and trustee of your slim body.

There are no handcuffs and no solitary confinement, unless you try to break out. Edward G. Robinson, James Cagney, and Gene Hackman won't sneak around and force-feed you pecan waffles with whipped butter and real maple syrup.

On the day after your Controlled Cheating Day, slap on your best slammer smile, pull on your form-fitting striped overalls, and calmly step behind the bars. (No whimpering allowed.) You can have visitors, but under no circumstances is there to be a file hidden in a Sara Lee German chocolate cake.

Confined in your Slimmer Slammer, there are criminal activities you will have to give up. You can't hold up a Baskin-Robbins for a pralines and cream cone or saw through a Big Mac with your teeth and expect to get away with it.

Buck up. The prison cafeteria has plenty for you to eat. You won't be on bread and water. You've got your Goldberg Eating Plan with hundreds of good food substitutions. As you're sitting behind bars peering out into the free eating world, don't despair; you're going to get sprung in a few days.

Keep staring at the Controlled Cheater's gorgeous heroine, the Statue of Liberty. Your day will come.

FATS GOLDBERG'S
DIET DAY EXERCISES FOR TEETH, GUMS, TONGUE, LIPS, CHEEKS, AND JAWS

These are specially designed exercises for Controlled Cheaters to use on Diet Days. Since you will not be strenuously using these six vitally important areas of your eating equipment every day, it is imper-

ative that they not get flabby or have spider webs form
from being underused.

You can exercise any time or place. I would ad-
vise, however, that you do not exercise in public places
because of other folks' severe questioning of your mental capabilities.

TOOTHPICK TUSSLE: Slide a round or flat
toothpick between each tooth. Whirl toothpick four
revolutions to the right, then six revolutions to the left,
or until you take off like a helicopter. If you are wealthy,
you may use Stim-U-Dents, interdental stimulators.

MOLAR MASH: This is an isometric exercise.
Slowly close molars on a small log like Fido fetching a
stick. Wag your tail, sit up, and beg for a treat. (But
you can't have it 'til your Cheating Day!)

*DENTAL FLOSS SLIDE WITH JAW MA-
NIPULATION:* Open jaw wide enough to get un-
restricted view of tonsils. Slide dental floss between
each tooth. If anything interesting comes out, like
orange pulp or spinach sprigs, be sure to save it for a
snack later on.

CHEEKS AND LIPS LIFT: Pucker lips and
suck cheeks toward teeth like you are slurping a vanilla malt through a straw. Make loud, rude, inhaling
sounds. This will come in handy if you are trying to
dry off your teeth or vacuuming the rug.

TIPPING THE SCALES

After you brush your teeth in the morning, take
off all your clothes and pull your pal, the scale, out of
its place of honor in the back of the closet and set it on
the favorite spot where you always weigh less. Jaunty-
jolly, step right up on the scale.

Before looking at the dial, smile as wide as you
can until the corners of your mouth are almost in your
eardrums. Then with courage and mighty resolve,

force your baby blues to look down and check where the needle stops. Whatever you do, do not scream out loud. Also, make sure your eyeballs don't fall out from surprise.

Many times after a Cheating Day, I think my eyes are playing tricks on me and I'm not reading the numbers right. I also stand on the scale longer, staring down to make absolutely sure the stupid scale is right. There are days I've almost missed lunch because my feet have been planted on the scale for such a long time. Then I think something is drastically wrong with the scale. THAT NUMBER COULDN'T BE RIGHT! After sticking my head under a cold shower, I become rational again.

You are, of course, going to see a weight gain. Maybe anywhere from one to six pounds, depending on how fast you could stuff it in.

You are going to feel lousy, frustrated, depressed, and you're going to want to throw your Controlled Cheating Diet, your scale, and me out of the window. You might even want to throw yourself after us. Hold on to the shower curtain for moral support if you get too close to the window. These are natural feelings. Who wouldn't get twitchy? You stuck to your diet like Elmer's Glue. You lost plenty of weight and then you went out and cheated one dirty, dumb, rotten day and you put back on three quarters of the weight you've struggled to take off.

Never you fret. These gloomy thoughts will soon go away and so will the added weight. I'll tell you how to get rid of both.

1. Surprise, surprise. You didn't really gain back all those tough pounds you've lost. Even you can't eat that much. Here you are after that wonderful Cheating Eating Day, and you're still ahead in the weight-loss game, because

you have six more days to lose those Cheating Day pounds and *even* more. So relax.

2. Controlled Cheating is a lifetime plan. You knew you were going to cheat, basically what you were going to eat, and probably how much. This is not a two-week diet you crash on and then go bozo and slap all the weight back on. This an eating program to follow the rest of your skinny days. It takes time. You have time. So relax.

3. You have a dynamite, low-fat, balanced diet to return to with all sorts of different foods to help you lose the pounds you've added back and then some. So relax.

4. As soon as you can get your eyes unglued from the scale, think back over yesterday, reliving every delicious bite and the hot time you had. Start from the moment your eyes flew open in the morning until you closed your food-heavy lids at night. So relax.

5. While your toes are still curled around the edge of the scale with terror, start thinking about your next Cheating Eating, only six short days away. This is not the end of your eating career, but the beginning. So relax.

As I'm sitting here typing on a beautiful June morning, the tears are falling down my cheeks. Yesterday was a Cheating Day for me, and today when I hopped on my Health-O-Meter, the few remaining hairs on my head stood on end. I had gained four pounds. Usually I can tell approximately how much I'm going to gain but I sure got fooled this time.

Sadness and anger poured out of every pore. Then I went through the Fabulous Five Feel-goods I just listed for you and now I feel better. Thanks.

LAUGH YOUR TUSH OFF.

YOU MUST GO BACK ON YOUR DIET
AND EXERCISE YOURSELF

There is absolutely no other way I can say it. I'm looking you straight in the eye and I'm telling you, straight from the shoulder, the truth.

YOU: That is Y-O-U. I'm saying you. Not the lady with the Sears shopping bag sitting next to you on the bus, or Ralph down the street, who's having a garage sale, or the husband of your Aunt Hilda. I'm talking to YOU.

MUST: That is M-U-S-T. No maybes, perhapses, or possiblies. MUST means there is no room for maneuvers or delays or tricks you've been playing on yourself. MUST is a command.

GO: G-O means to move. Move to your diet. Not sideways or at an angle. That's a straight line to your low-calorie, balanced diet. I'm waiting.

BACK: B-A-C-K means to return to the program, to the diet program that you used the last two weeks. You are returning, but at the same time what you are actually doing is moving forward. You are moving forward because you will begin losing weight again and continuing your march to your Goal Weight. *Back*, in this case, means full speed ahead.

ON: O-N means following the diet to the letter. You are *On* top of the diet. Not underneath, to the sides, or around the back where you can cheat.

YOUR: Y-O-U-R is the possessive form of you. This is *Your* diet and it's going to give you the form you want to possess. No one is going to knock on your door and tell you they can lose the weight for you. No one else can lose weight and keep it off for you.

DIET: D-I-E-T means the specific weight loss program outlined for you.

Spelling it out once more for you kids in the back row:

Y-O-U M-U-S-T G-O B-A-C-K
O-N Y-O-U-R D-I-E-T.

ONE DAY AT A TIME

That's right. Do everything in this book one day at a time. Today is *the* day. The only day in our lives. Yesterday is "Gone With The Wind," and you can't see tomorrow lurking around the corner, unless you have long eyeballs. We can do absolutely nothing about yesterday. Like that pound and a half of onion rings you ate four years ago, it's all ancient history.

Regardless of what your horoscope predicts about meeting someone tall, dark, and rich, you can't tell what's going to happen tomorrow. So why worry and stew about how many days you have to eat iceberg lettuce before you can cheat again? Diet for today *only*!

When it's a Controlled Cheating Day, enjoy that glorious day to the fullest extent of the holes in your belt. Laugh, sing, dance, cavort, eat. Don't start thinking in the middle of the afternoon about tomorrow when you have to go back on your dumb diet.

Forget yesterday and tomorrow. Live for today. Today is the only twenty-four hours we've got for sure.

HARK! LOOK! LISTEN! HEAR YE! HEAR YE!

The A Number One accomplishment of my thirty-two years of losing weight and keeping it off is the ability to go back on my diet immediately, the very day after a Controlled Cheating Day.

I know, I know. You're sick of this one thought, but I have to keep coming back to it for your sake and mine. *There are no secrets to losing weight and keeping it off.* You'd better get used to this idea because I'm going to come back to it many more times.

If there is one idea, thought, practice, or method

that comes close to magic in controlling weight, this is it—the ability to go back on your diet after a Controlled Cheating Day.

Controlled Cheating's success is based on this one principle. This is the guiding light, the royal flush, and the big payoff. *The one reason why I have been successful in losing weight (and you can be, too) is my ability to go back on the diet without hemming and hawing or hesitation after I've cheated. Nothing else counts.*

Controlled Cheating is the release. Going back on the diet is the "key." Sometimes the key is hard to turn and you have to force it, but the door that opens is your Open Sesame to slim freedom and happiness.

From my earliest memories, I've been obsessed with losing weight and dieting. I bought every diet book published and went to the best diet doctors in Kansas City. I talked to friends and enemies alike. I cussed. I screamed. I prayed. I tore at my clothes. Finally some kind soul would throw a bucket of cold Pepsi-Cola on me and I would return to reality. And try to find another diet that would work. That was my reality, my avocation, my full-time job.

The saga, pre-age twenty-five, was always the same. I would get every doctor's diet, diet-book diet, or a diet from a passing bus driver. I would go on the dumb diet, stick to it for a few days, or maybe even a week or two, then I would cheat. It didn't have to be one full day. If I just ate three cinnamon rolls in two minutes, I was gone again. The diet was busted and I rolled out eating faster and harder than ever.

This went on for years. The same vicious circle. I would start dieting, cheat for one minute, and be off and stuffing it in nonstop for another four months.

In 1957, I was waiting tables at my fraternity house, Zeta Beta Tau, at the University of Missouri. I waited tables because I could eat all I wanted. One lunch I'll never forget: three complete lunches, total-

ing six greasy cheeseburgers, a gallon of cold apple-
sauce, and a pound of potato chips, plus four chunky
peanut-butter-and-jelly sandwiches loaded with margarine, two quarts of milk, and three pieces of chocolate cake.

Struggling up the steps from the kitchen, I thought
the end was near. I willed my size-50 khaki pants to
Dumbo the elephant. I had been stuffed before but
nothing ever like this. I lay down on the floor, out of
breath and moaning, until a fraternity brother took
pity on me and drove me over to the student infirmary.
I got the head doctor at the infirmary to see me. I told
him what I had done and whimpered and pleaded for a
diet. He looked up through his bushy eyebrows and
(I'll never forget his words) said: "Don't eat so much."
Brilliant. As soon as he said that, I got hungry again.

Of course, he was the last doctor I saw for several
years. Back to the vicious circle. There was absolutely
no way on God's green earth that I could cheat on a diet
and then go back on that diet. It didn't work. Every
diet I found operated like a crash diet. I was always
bailing out.

The reason was simple. I didn't know what I was
doing. There was no plan to follow. I didn't have control. I wasn't organizing my body to diet by feeding it
what it needed while denying it what it didn't.

Finally, I figured out Controlled Cheating for myself. Cheating has been with us since dieting began,
when Cindy and Clyde Cavepersons couldn't fit into
their dinosaur-skin bikinis. Since cheating couldn't be
avoided or abolished, there had to be a way to make it
fit into my scheme of things, to make it work for, not
against, the diet.

As any good burglar knows, a lock must release to
work smoothly. The dieting key is the desire and need
to go back on the diet. Controlled Cheating works

smoothly because you have your Cheating Days to provide the release for that all-important key.

Everyone who diets is going to cheat. As sure as there isn't enough chocolate in the world, people on diets are going to cheat. Then after they cheat, the guilt, bad feelings, and food depression set in. Every other fatty will scream at the heavens, "What's the use! I just can't do it. I'm weak and nothing but a fat slob."

To go on a diet that never gives you the opportunity to cheat is not realistic. Not only that, it's a pie in the face of what overweight human beings actually do. It's an insult to us.

The main reason why people can't lose weight and keep it off is that they can't go back on their diet once they cheat. Controlled Cheating totally eliminates that problem. You and I have our Controlled Cheating Days and cheating is built into our lives. No guilt, no depression afterward. We need it, we deserve it, and, with Fats Goldberg, we get it!

H₂O, HO, HO, HO

Water works for me. You can bet your bottom ice cube it will lubricate your body too.

I've been drinking at least ten eight-ounce glasses of tap water every day since forever. Originally I started slurping because I was thirsty and good old water filled me up (temporarily) with NO CALORIES.

Finally I found out how healthy H_2O is plus how crucial water is to lose those pounds and keep them off.

GOLDBERG'S GURGLING GUIDE

- Drink at least eight to ten eight-ounce glasses of water every day, including your Cheating Day.
- Keep a glass of water handy wherever you are.
- Pour six to eight glasses of water in a container and pour from that.
- Try drinking in pairs—with your sweetie pie, or two glasses at a time.

- Get one of those plastic jugs with the straw attached and carry it around with you on your hip, and maybe you could become Wyatt Slurp, the fastest water drinker in the West.

WORDS OF WONDER ABOUT WATER

- Water is our most important nutrient.
- Water makes up about 55 percent of our body weight.
- Water helps our bods metabolize stored fat.
- The best perscription to get rid of fluid retention is, surprise, drink more water!
- Water gets rid of waste and helps relieve constipation.
- Water greases up the joints and everything else.
- Cold water is absorbed into your body faster than warm water.
- You might think you're going to float away, but it's almost impossible to drink too much water. Our bodies get rid of excess water. So keep slurping.
- You must drink *more* cold water before, during, and after exercising.
- Water helps to keep the body temperature constant, like an air conditioner.
- We can live only a few days without water. Without food, we can live about two months.
- Ice water does not cause cramps. Gulping water in a hurry causes stomach problems.
- Water helps us breathe. It keeps our lungs moist.
- Our skin looks and feels healthier when we drink water. You should see my rosy cheeks.
- Here's a news flash for you: Water is in all our drinks. There's plenty of water in everything

we eat too, especially fruits and vegetables. They contain more than 80 percent water.

- If you don't keep your muscles pumped up with water, you'll feel weak and tired.
- Water carries nutrients to all parts of the body.
- Squirt some fresh lime or lemon juice in your water for a tasty treat.
- Try drinking with a straw to keep your lips puckered.
- Drink plain water instead of soda pop, coffee, or tea.
- Water is great for the kidneys and reduces the risk of kidney stones.
- Always know the location of the bathroom wherever you are. Hotels always have plenty of bathrooms. If you spot a drinking fountain, you can be fairly sure there is a bathroom nearby. Don't wait until the last minute.

BOTTLED WATERS

Tap water straight out of the faucet is my favorite. I'm too cheap to buy water in those funny looking bottles.

But to give you the whole picture of this water business, let me explain the differences:

1. *Seltzer or 2% Plain:* Tap water that is filtered and made fizzy with carbon dioxide.
2. *Club Soda:* Artifically carbonated tap water with added sodium and minerals.
3. *Mineral Water:* Water that has natural or added minerals.
4. *Distilled Water:* Water that is boiled, turned into steam which leaves all the impurities behind, then recondensed back into water. When I was sixteen, I drove a '37 Oldsmobile. Cousin

Dave Gelhaar had a gas station across the street. He told me to use distilled water in my battery. I'll let *you* drink distilled water. I'm afraid I might light up.

5. *Sparkling Water:* Any natural or artificially carbonated water.

6. *Spring Water:* Water that springs out of the earth, untampered with, and is bottled nearby.

There are hundreds of bottled waters. Check those labels for everything, especially for sodium and salts.

I'm so thirsty, my tongue is hanging out. Excuse me, my faucet is running.

SLIMAGERY

HOW TO LAUGH YOUR TUSH OFF
AND
OTHER HEADY SUBJECTS

I was looking around for a word that could nail down the interaction between the body and mind when we want to lose weight and keep it off.

Slimagery!

Our imaginations are miraculous. We can picture anything; losing thirty pounds, seeing our necks again, eating a raft of Ben and Jerry's ice cream, buttoning our pants without getting a hernia, dating the best looking babe (man or woman) at the office, or anything the heart desires.

Imagination is like a muscle. Your imagination can be so full of ideas, it is strong, hard, and bursting out of its T-shirt. Or it can be flabby, weak, and have barely enough strength to turn on the TV and stare at reruns of "The Rockford Files." The more we use our imaginations the stronger they get. USE YOUR POSITIVE ENERGY TO EXERCISE THE MIND LIKE YOU DO YOUR BODY.

Now don't start whining, "I don't have any imagination." That's a load of brussels sprouts (or worse). You can think, therefore you've got an imagination, and it's powerful.

We think in pictures. I'm an Olympic daydreamer myself. Let me tell you, I can conjure up some hot pictures. This is also called mental rehearsals, or "mind movies."

As much as we all love to watch movies, eventually we have to put down the bag of buttered popcorn and start to move. Which brings me back to good old Controlled Cheating.

We can fantasize our whole lives about losing weight, feeling peppy, wearing sharp clothes, or any other of the millions of dreams that race through our minds. But eventually, we have to stop procrastination and start moving.

I believe in *positive* action. Haul your bod out of that recliner. Take a walk. Put down that Snickers. Do something.

First we think, then we do. The way to learn Controlled Cheating is to *do* Controlled Cheating.

Ah, when you see those pounds flying to the Fat Bank, and you look at the new you, your whole life will change. You've done something positive for yourself, and that positiveness will invigorate your imagination. Miracles *will* happen.

Take the girdle off your imagination. Let it soar. Then do something with it. Anything that works to lose weight is good. Yell at the moon. Meditate. Become a ventriloquist. Walk a marathon. Raise llamas. Play the drums. Run for mayor.

Imagination leads to action. Slimagery is a learned skill, like riding a bicycle. Even if you fall off, you can scramble back on. And you can use your slimagination to take you wherever you want to go.

HOW TO LAUGH YOUR TUSH OFF
THE SLIMAGERY WAY

1. Set your Goal Weight. Brand that number on your imagination.
2. Keep a clear picture of your slim body at your Goal Weight.
3. Run movies through your mind of eating healthy, nutritious foods, giggling as you walk with your sweetie, and drinking delicious water.
4. Visualize eating every morsel of grease, dough, and sugar on your Cheating Day.
5. Laugh as you see those pounds drop off your body forever.
6. There are lots of ways to laugh. Here are some Goldberg Giggle Variations to get you started:

LAUGH YOUR TUSH OFF

LAUGH: It's the best exercise and you don't need Nikes.

GIGGLE: It stretches certain muscles and will make you glow down to your toes.

GUFFAW: As you picture yourself a thin person, completely in control of your mouth and life, no longer a prisoner, fighting to get out of a bag of nacho-flavored Doritos.

CHORTLE: While you think about the new slim you.

SMILE: At your self-confidence, sense of accomplishment, party-going, and the tight T-shirts you can wear.

GRIN: Knowing you are wonderful already and that losing weight and keeping it off will only improve a good life.

CHUCKLE: Your body will laugh with relief
              from getting rid of that excess fat.
SNICKER: To yourself and know deep down
              nothing can stop you from reaching
              your goal.

NAGGING

Nagging is a nasty word. I've been nagged by experts most of my natural life. Nagging is the most negative thing you can do to an overweight person. Even looking at the way the letters fit together shows it's a truly foul word. Nagging gets my blood as hot as pizza cheese.

Fat people get nagged more than anyone else alive because their problem is right out there for everyone to see. We chubbies are large, hard-to-miss targets, so we're easy prey for every loudmouth. The earliest memories I have are of other kids teasing, kidding, and making fun of how fat I was. You know what they used to sing: "Fatty, fatty, two by four, couldn't get through the streetcar door."

The teasing went on until I could grab their skinny little bodies and sit on their legs. Eventually I developed a fast mouth and could give back the kidding with even more knives attached. Shoot, I didn't win anything doing that either.

In all my experience, nagging, slamming, rapping, criticizing, or ragging has never gotten an overweight person to lose weight and keep it off. Nagging works exactly in the opposite way. What actually happens is that we fatties eat even more from anger and to show those gatemouths what we can really do.

Something I cannot understand about naggers (*we* are the *nagees*) is that they cannot get the idea through their stupid heads that *we know* we're fat. Naggers think they're giving us this brand-new piece of news hot off the wires. You bet we know we're fat. All it takes is a scalding case of heartburn and a quick glance in the mirror to see our bulging clothes—our constant reminders.

To their credit, naggers sincerely think they are helping us. What they don't understand is that the way to really help us is to leave us alone, or else sit down with us and try to understand where we are in our Battle of the Bulge.

God bless my folks. They never nagged or criticized. Their leaving me alone was one of the main reasons why I eventually lost weight and kept it off. They let me figure it out for myself. They had confidence in me.

The only time I ever heard anything from my folks was occasionally when I was working in the market and I had my whole head, instead of just one hand, buried in a big box of Nabisco vanilla sandwich cookies. They would just say, "Larry!" But that didn't stop me either.

Naggers come in all forms. They can be parents, brothers, sisters, friends, relatives, teachers—people who honestly do like you. Regardless, the results are always the same, a big *zero*.

Naggers feel they're superior to us. To their thin minds, all we need is a *little* push, a *little* yelling, a *little* nudge and we'll straighten out and become thin and perfect—just like them. If only it were that easy.

Naggers are always experts on other people's problems, whether it's overeating, or over or under anything else. No wonder they call old, beat-up, rundown horses *nags*. Why don't naggers nag *themselves* into faultless, flawless human beings? Who asked for their advice anyway? There are certain people I go to when I want advice. I trust their intelligence and judgment, and I ask for it.

There's a great quote I remember when I get

unwanted advice and guidance: "If you can tell good advice from bad advice, you don't need advice." (With free advice, you get what you pay for.)

Now, the same people who nagged me when I was fat are still nagging "You're much too thin. You could afford to put on a few pounds. We can see your bones!" I can never win, except with the folks that count with me.

People nagging at you won't help; you have to help yourself to dieting. But if the naggers are folks you otherwise like or have to live with, you'll just have to grit your teeth and put up with it . . . for a while. If the naggers won't stop, give it back to them with both barrels, with plenty of kidding and teasing about their weaknesses. Do it with a smile and make them laugh. The best defense is a good jolly offense.

The sole purpose of this book is to get you to reexamine your lives and eating habits and understand there is a way to lose weight and keep it off and still be a happy eater.

I promise I'll never nag you about it.

LIKE YOURSELF

I like "like." Love is a nice word, but it sort of falls out of your mouth. Say "love" and your jaw drops open, your tongue looks like a soggy washcloth, and love dribbles out. *Like* has a fresh, crisp sound, and you can hardly say it without smiling.

I like myself. I'm my own best pal. When I started dieting, I didn't like myself. Folks wrote me off as another fat guy who couldn't keep his hand out of the groceries. My self-esteem was lower than the last drop of Heinz ketchup in the bottle.

My first big break came when the *Chicago Tribune* gave me a job in 1958. There I was, over 325 big ones, one suit (which I couldn't button), a 1951 pea-green Pontiac, a bag of stale bagels, and six warm Pepsis. But the *Chicago Tribune* liked me. That made me feel terrific. They had confidence and accepted me for what I was. That made me want to be better.

I didn't understand all this in 1958, but I started dieting. I was plain tired of being fat, so I began losing weight. Looking in the mirror at my vanishing body and buttoning my pants with ease, I began to like myself more.

Then other people noticed and started yelling about how good I looked. A few took me aside and asked how I was doing it. My diet plan was just starting to take shape—like me. The more I lost, the better I felt about myself. The better I felt about myself, the more my family and friends gave me a pat on the buns. The more patting, the smaller the buns.

The whole thing is a big wondrous circle that you can jump into anytime, too. Look inside yourself. Look outside yourself. You're going to like what you see.

THE FIRST HURRAH

Everyone, including you, needs a cheering section: a warm body you can talk to when your stomach feels as empty as the Grand Canyon, when you get discouraged, depressed, and want to nuke the whole diet idea.

Depend on your family, friends, or just one good pal. You can call them any time of the day or night. Get everything out on the table. Maybe scream and yell. They'll give you an encouraging word, I promise.

RELAX AND TAKE IT EASY

Sit back, take off your saddle shoes, prop your feet up with the holes in the socks, loosen your belt (you might have to anyway), scratch wherever it itches, and relax. You're about to start on a long tour, because I want you to live to be 120 and happy.

Controlled Cheating is a lifetime tap dance. Because it is a plan that lasts the rest of your life, being twitchy, tense, nervous, irritable, and an all 'round nudge won't work. Besides, folks won't want to hang out with you. You must learn to relax and take it easy. *Do not* take yourself too seriously.

None of us is perfect and you're going to make mistakes. And you're going to make errors that will cost you rotten, filthy pounds. I still make mistakes, plenty of them. At times, I feel I can play my body like a 150-pound Stradivarius strumming the Minute Waltz. But on any Diet Day, I can eat all the right foods, get plenty of exercise, do everything right, and *pow,* eat something stupid that I think is low calorie and, of course, it isn't.

Hopping on the scale the next morning, I scream with terror. That dumb needle didn't move down, and even worse, I slapped on a pound.

Over the years, I've learned to say over and over in the relaxer section of my brain, which is right next to the panic button, relax, relax, *relax.* The more you take it easy and relax, the more energy you'll have for dieting.

I also cool it by singing, whistling, and talking to myself. Sometimes I even do it out loud, which is fine if you're in New York, because most folks talk to themselves out loud anyway—and nobody notices.

TALKING TO THE BIG PERSON

Yeah, I pray. Prayer makes me feel good. Being Jewish, most of my organized prayer has been in synagogues. But I've done some heavy-duty praying in Catholic, Baptist, Congregational, you name it, churches.

My personal belief is that God is everywhere and has a great sense of humor. Maybe God has a weight problem too. If I want to talk to Him or Her, I can be eating a juicy sirloin and buttery hash browns, kissing a lady, walking, flying white-knuckled on an airplane, or anywhere. I do plenty of praying on airplanes. Deep down, I'm an evangelist, a slim evangelist, preaching the joys of a normal, slim life. (I'll deliver my Sermon on the Mounds at the end of the book.)

Prayer can work for you. It's the best and cheapest do-it-yourself mental health. You'll be amazed at the number of hunger pains God can take away.

I pray almost every night after Johnny Carson and before I go to sleep. I thank God for the day, for keeping me lean, and for keeping my family and pals safe. Then I pass God all my problems, ask for a good day tomorrow, roll over, and dream of chocolate doughnuts.

GOAL WEIGHT: ANOTHER EATS DAY

THE ENVELOPE PLEASE. YOU HAVE WON "THE CHEATER," A COMBINATION OF THE OSCAR, TONY, EMMY, AND GRAMMY OF DIETING!!! HURRAY!! HURRAH!! CONGRATULATIONS!!

The winner of the coveted Cheater Award for Best Performance in Controlled Cheating is YOU.

Run to your kitchen where The Cheater Award is always presented, clutch it, choke back a tear of happiness, and gush, "Thank you. Thank you, everyone. There are so many wonderful people I'd like to thank. First: me, myself, and I. Second: the producers—my mother and father. Third: the writer, the director, and the person in charge of the refreshment stand, yours truly."

The Cheater statuette is a beautiful, simulated alligator-covered garbage disposal with a hole wide enough to slide in a ten-inch cherry pie without crumbling the crust.

The Cheater is not to be taken lightly. It shows you have stamina, wisdom, strength, and most important, you're an all 'round good person who's reached your Goal Weight with Controlled Cheating. You, award winner, have reached your Goal Weight and earned the votes, plaudits, and accolades (that's different than lemonades) of the eighty million dieters in the United States.

Take a close peek at your award and you'll see that the last five letters of "Cheater" spell Eater! Being an award-winning Cheater shows that you are a smart Eater.

Congratulations!

Knowing you, you've already thumbed through this book and seen that your swiftly slimming silhouette can afford another Controlled Cheating Day.

Yes! Your mind and body can now handle an extra goody day because you've got your Controlled Cheating batting swing in a great low-cal groove.

Good ol' dieting, like good ol' baseball, has become the national pastime. But losing weight and keeping it off is more toil than a pleasant afternoon in the Wrigley Field bleachers getting a beautiful tan, an icy beer in one hand, juicy hot dog with plenty of yellow mustard in the other, and two bags of peanuts roasting in your lap. By now you know dieting is a full-time job. Every day while you are either applying your makeup or scraping those tough whiskers off your face, you must also go right to work on your Controlled Cheating.

Look at it this way. It's your business. You're the head honcho, boss, supervisor, foreman, union, and only employee. We Controlled Cheaters take our orders from a whole raft of barking bosses all screaming from the inside of our own beautiful skins. Cheating Eating is no eight-hour-a-day job, either. It's twenty-four hours a day, six days a week—and no doughnut and coffee breaks (except on those you-know-when days).

You've already got one day off, and now because you've been such a loyal and hard worker you can take another day off. Hooray! And you didn't even have to go on strike. That's some good job.

Don't go nuts from all the excitement. There's no retirement from the job. No gold watch. No little house on the coast of Florida where you can grow your own orange soda pop and watch the sun set over the top of your Lorna Doones.

What you get is a life of good health and thinness. Controlled Cheating is the best job in the world. You're in business for yourself. And yourself is the business. All the decisions and rewards are yours. Controlled Cheating is a good time. And who wants to retire from a good time, anyway?

Controlled Cheating didn't come down from the sky all of a sudden three fast decades ago on a butter-flavored golden beam to bathe me in its spectacular light. I had no idea what I was doing. I *did* know that what I had been doing the first twenty-five years of my life wasn't working. I knew I had to cheat. That was a fat fact of life—my life.

I also knew that what I was doing was working. I didn't call it Controlled Cheating until 1961 or 1962. I didn't call it controlled or even cheating. I called it, "I get to eat everything on Sundays."

What I did decide was that it was better to cheat on one day rather than all seven. Also, it was better to live with one day of eating what I wanted to, with good sense, rather than no days of fun food. I could finally lose weight and keep it off on my program. It was better to control and plan what I was doing rather than shooting up and down all the time like an express elevator in the Empire State Building.

During the first year of my diet, during 1959 and 1960, when I dropped from over 325 to 190, I thought the only time God was going to allow me to eat my precious goodies was one lonely day a week.

The thought never flashed through my curly head that someday I would be able to cheat twice a week. One day a week was okay. I was almost normal weight, 175 pounds, happy, in good health, and had enough energy to rassle with a grizzly.

All of sudden in 1968, I was in Goldberg's Pizzeria business, standing in front of two 650-degree roaring ovens for ten hours a day schlepping pizzas. Boy, that needle on the old Health-O-Meter whizzed down like my body was in a severe economic recession. One sunny Sunday morning the scale shouted 160. Joyfully, prancing off the scale, the spectacular thought hit me that maybe, just maybe, I could cheat twice a week.

At first I told myself, "Nah, you can't do that, Goldberg. You've been slim for twelve years and all of a sudden you want to fool around with success. You must be some kind of a dieting dummy. You're going to be off and eating like the old days. Why blow ten years of the good thin life?"

But I couldn't stop it. The glorious thought of two Cheating Days kept whizzing through my brain. Naturally, being a fat man disguised as a thin man, what else would I think about?

I stuck one hand in the mozzarella cheese and the other in the pepperoni. This was how I did my best meditating. I made the decision.

Mumbling to myself, which frightened two customers enough for them to bolt out the door dragging their half-eaten mushroom pizza with them, I said, "Look, big boy, you've done a great job for the last twelve years. The chances of you going out of control are 'slim.' If this doesn't work, you haven't lost a thing. You can always go back to one Cheating Day a week. Big deal. Give it a shot."

In those days, I closed the pizza store on Mondays. Of course, I cheated on Mondays. I also took Thursday nights off. Thursdays would be the natural time to add the Cheating Day. I could have another hot date, and there were still two or three days in between to lose the weight I would gain on Thursdays and Mondays.

I tried it and I liked it. My body and mind said thanks, too. I didn't shoot up and start gaining again as I feared. I even lost another ten pounds.

With either two or three days between Controlled Cheating Days, I found I easily lost the weight I added on those days. I became smarter in my cheating, lived a more normal life, and I learned to "double my pleasure and double my fun."

But I was still rigid about my Cheating Days; only Mondays and Thursdays, for five more years. When I started franchising my pizza places, I had Saturdays and Sundays off. Saturday would be a great day to cheat. I could have a Saturday night date (if I could find one). There were more rip-roaring social events on Saturdays and I could have half a weekend for some giggles.

Fear reared its ugly tummy. I was afraid to change those days from Monday and Thursday to Wednesday and Saturday. Still, after fifteen solid years of Controlled Cheating, I was quaking in my size 11D boots, afraid I was going to blow my thinness. You've probably already got the crystal-clear message that it takes me a long time to change. At least when it comes to Controlled Cheating.

Sticking one hand in the pizza dough and the other in the anchovies (I changed my meditating spots, too), I said, "Full mouth ahead." Changing the Cheating Days worked out fine.

So in thirty-two years of Controlled Cheating Eating, I have changed my program only two times. Deep down, this was fine with me; when it comes to losing weight and keeping it off, slow and steady is best.

YOUR CONTROLLED CHEATING DAYS MUST BE TWO OR THREE DAYS APART. THEY CAN NEVER BE TWO DAYS IN A ROW.

Most folks are off Saturday and Sunday. I know what you're thinking: Those days sure would be ideal to cheat. Back off now. Two days in a row are dangerous even if they're Wednesday and Thursday.

1. Two straight Cheating Eating Days will give you too big a weight gain, not to mention a third-degree case of heartburn. This will make you twitchy, depressed, and frustrated. You might get so nervous you'll blow the whole program and sprint toward uncontrolled cheating. Fat City, here you come again. Too many cheeseburgers with grilled onions is too big a load for your slimming mind and body. There would be too many lines on the scale that would have to be lost.
2. Splitting the two days will let your body and mind lose the pounds you've gained so easily.
3. When you break up the days, you can mess up on Cheating Day and you still have another big day a couple of steps down the road. "Messing Up" means eating stupid, empty, high-calorie foods you didn't genuinely crave. You ate them because it was a Cheating Day and you had a couple of empty hands.

I've done this about two thousand times in my Cheating Eating life. There I am, on my day, no diet, no date, no social event, just standing there with nothing to do but eat. And I run around eating ridiculous stuff only because I can do it all day. I pile on foods that don't get me truly excited.

For instance, gallons of high-calorie soda that give me no food fix but dull the appetite with empty calories. Then I move on to those terrible gummy little supermarket cakes, maybe a cold hot dog on a bun that was baked for the soldiers in the War of 1812. Or I drop in a grease pit where I know the food would turn off a trash compactor.

I don't have to be alone, either. I could be at someone's house for a lousy dinner or go out with pals and get bad eats plus spending a Brink's truck full of money. A double whammy. A wasted day. But it's isolated. No next day to compound the damage. Instead, immediate retraction. And wait till the next Cheating Day for the guilt to recede.

The feeling I want you to have as you tuck yourself in at the end of a Cheating Day is the pleasant glow of eating satisfaction. Before you close your eyes, you drift back over the day and smile that there wasn't one wasted calorie.

The next morning you'll hop on the scale and grin because those couple of pounds you gained were worth it. You go back to your low-calorie balanced diet with no regrets and a quick takeoff and additional loss.

4. With the Cheating Days split up, you always have something great to look forward to. Instead of one distant light of eating at the end of a long, low-calorie tunnel, you have two bright lights in two short blocks. You'll feel good.

SECRETS: BOZO EATING

Bozo or nutsy or crazy eating is ramming, jamming, stuffing, sliding, and maneuvering all the delicious goodies you can get into your mouth at the same time. You do this whether you're hungry or not, and you go bozo only because it's a Cheating Day. Deep down you feel that you must get as much food as you can behind your cute little navel, because tomorrow is a Diet Day.

Ah, you've been a good, top-flight Controlled Cheater for a while now, and you have gotten this wonderful feeling that crazy, bozo hogging-it-up eating doesn't always satisfy you. Hold on: The truth is that eating only when you're hungry is much more satisfying and fun.

It only took me fifteen years to finally discover why my Controlled Cheating Days weren't quite doing the job. I discovered that if I waited until I was good and hungry, I had a better time than when I ate solely because I could with no guilt or restrictions.

In my early Cheating Eating Days, I used to start chewing even if I had nothing in my mouth. The teeth were going up and down and sideways even when I was only a quarter inch below that completely stuffed open-the-top-button feeling.

It makes no difference whether you want to eat a pretzel with yellow mustard or lobster tails with a quart of drawn butter. When you genuinely want to eat and you're hungry, you are going to enjoy what you're eating 1,000 percent more than when you're so full the tacos are inching out of your ears.

MYSTERY

I love a mystery. Everyone gets all tingly when skeletons fall out of corn cob-webbed closets, or gnarly, bacon-greased hands come out from behind chocolate-brown velvet drapes and circle the beautiful neck of a screaming cook who forgot to put the fresh bread on the table when she laid out the chunky peanut butter and grape jelly.

One mystery that scares me and makes me laugh the most is discovering something that I didn't know about my skinny body.

A mystery that always baffles me is, on Controlled Cheating Days, when I decided to eat only when I got hungry, several wonderful things happened:

1. My eating habits became more normal. Now I know that the way I eat will never become normal like the born skinnies eat. However, my normal is a heck of an improvement over the way I used to eat.
2. I actually eat less.
3. I have a better time and more fun than when I hoist in the goodies like a steam shovel.

Why a former fatty like me, who lives to eat, who would kill for a cashew, and who on a Diet Day has a constant edge of being hungry, can have a giggling Cheating Day by eating only foods that I truly ache for is a mystery. When I eat only my favorite grease, dough, and sugar, my Cheating Day is so much better than one on which I eat like an unclogged drain in my kitchen sink.

Sure the body must change. I don't know how or why. I haven't lost the constant urge to eat, but I have become rational in my eating. Hooray for big favors, little favors, and Oreos.

Your body will change, too. With Controlled Cheating you will listen more to your body and feel what it wants and doesn't want. You'll also feel terrific mentally and physically now that you have a natural control over your eating.

Ah, sugar-sweet mystery of life.

SURPRISE

You'll become more relaxed about your eating on your Diet Days and Cheating Eating Days.

With two Cheating Days, there isn't the constant pressure of only one special day, when you sprint out of the house so ravenous, you'd munch on the dandelions sprouting between the cracks in the sidewalk until you can get to your local doughnut store.

Waking up, you'll take a long, luxurious, relaxing stretch and realize that you have a terrific Controlled Cheating Day ahead of you. Don't get frightened. Cheating Days will never become a bore. There will always be that air of excitement and electricity. Folks on the bus will stare because your head will gleam like a 250-watt bulb. But you'll have a relaxed glow.

The basic rules of controlled eating on the Diet Days will not change. For us former fatties, eternal vigilance is and must be our constant companion. With the extra Cheating Day, you will become more relaxed, which will make you stronger because now you know that you can lose weight and keep it off permanently.

Surprise: You never thought it could happen.

A LITTLE FLEXIBILITY PLEASE

Now that you've reached two fabulous Cheating Days a week, you're a tough enough low-cal cookie to have a little flexibility. Flexibility? For what? By moving your hands to your mouth all these years, you've got more elbow flexibility than a major league pitcher. Flexibility about Cheating Days.

You can switch your Cheating Days. But remember. Always and always. Forever and ever. You *cannot* have two Controlled Cheating Days in a row. Consecutive is a four letter word (or it should be). You must be very careful switching Cheating Days. Aren't I simply marvelous? So good to you!

Suppose you originally chose Sunday and Thursday and now you want to change the days to Wednesday and Saturday. You cannot cheat on Thursday and again on Saturday. You can, dear dieter, cheat on Sunday and then cheat again on Wednesday to start your new Cheating Day schedule.

When it comes to switching, don't give yourself more than two Cheating Days in the transition week and think that neither your scale nor I will know the difference. We will. We always will.

After all the tummy-to-tummy conversations we've had, you know as well as I do the reasons for my, and yours, being this tough. But let's go over it again for those of you in the second balcony who couldn't hear all the lines.

1. Having less than two days between Cheating Eating Days doesn't give your body enough time to lose the weight you've gained. This is lethal for you physically and mentally.

2. If you continually mess around with your Cheating Days, you'll lose the set routine and guess what? Big Person's Shops, here you come again.

3. Flexibility doesn't mean anything goes. It says that now you can use your free will, sort of. Most of all,

YOU MUST GO BACK TO YOUR DIET!

As you're licking your finger to turn the page, guess what's coming? You're right!

YOU MUST GO BACK ON YOUR DIET!

Cheat as hard and as fast as you can, but after any Cheating Day,

YOU

MUST

GO

BACK

ON

YOUR

DIET,

BABY!

AFTER ANY CHEATING DAY.

YOUR BODY CHANGES

How do you like your new body? Looks good. You fit into jeans you haven't been able to button in six years. You've not only lost pounds but inches, too. The little economy car you bought finally fits without giving you a ridge in your stomach from the steering wheel. Your shoes are even flopping around your feet. You didn't know you could lose weight in your toes, did you? Your glasses rest on your nose, not on your cheeks.

Friends keep yelling, "Boy, do you look terrific. How much did you lose? Wish I could lose weight."

You're now a certifiable skinny. That's the outside of your body, the part everyone can see and that gives you such great pleasure. Bask in the glory; you deserve it.

A new you has emerged from your heavy overcoat of fat. By now you know that losing weight and keeping it off starts from the inside and works its way out.

You start by doing. Dieting is doing; it is an active verb. Don't start by trying to analyze everything you do before, during, and after you eat. If you do, you'll waste all your time trying to go deep into the recesses of your mind while your hand is going deeper into the bag of nacho-flavored Doritos.

Self-analysis is important and this comes as you're dieting, losing weight, and keeping it off. Every day that you're alive, new ideas, insights, and revelations will come to you naturally. Folks who keep analyzing without doing anything are copping out. They're waiting for that great beam from the sky to take them away to a skinny never-never land. In losing weight and keeping it off, *you learn by doing.*

Right now you're at the weight you want to be. You've probably learned more about yourself during this Controlled Cheating period than ever before.

Maybe now you can understand why you got fat in the first place, why you kept eating, and how you're going to stay at your Goal Weight.

Every day of the thirty-two years I've been Cheating Eating, I've learned something new about myself. Sometimes it comes in little bits and pieces that accumulate until I get the whole idea.

Over the last several years my tastes have changed. My craving for food is still the same and I'm still as hungry as before, but my desire for sugary foods has gone down. I suspect I've developed more sophisticated tastes, that want a variety of foods, not just the same old jelly-roll standbys of my youth. Ten years ago, I would have given you a lifetime of pizzas if you'd have told me that was going to happen. Oh sure, I still love ice cream, cakes, pies, and anything else with a sweet taste, but what I want even more on my Controlled Cheating Days are things like pasta, all different kinds of bread and butter, cheeses, fried chicken, steak, and chili. And all sorts of new, never-before-experienced restaurants: Argentinean, Czechoslovakian, Spanish, and Japanese. I want to experiment and enjoy it all.

Where you are now, a Controlled Cheater who has reached Goal Weight, is a wonderful coordination of mind and body that has proven that you can do most anything you want in life.

What's left of you deserves a big hug.

DIET DON'TS

You're the real thing, the genuine article. You've reached your Goal Weight and you're worthy of a mountain of congratulatory telegrams, ovations, cheers, and tributes. (And raviolis.)

Beware, Goal Weighter, of Diet Don'ts. I must warn you about these. They're obnoxious habits that will plunge your popularity to the level of a vacation weekend at a Siberian work camp.

Time to confess. I used to be guilty of all these offenses. That's why I know them so well. If you check yourself before you begin, it might save you many Saturday nights home alone.

THE DIET SNOB

A former fatty who swaggers down the street with an air of superiority looking down at folks who are overweight. Diet Snobs say to themselves, "Look at those fat slobs who can't control themselves. See that one at the soda fountain with the root beer float and the slice of chocolate cream pie.

He's not as self-disciplined or as wonderfully thin as I am." A Diet Snob scolds, huffs, and puffs about other people who can't control themselves. Remember, Goal Weighter, you're only one step away from Fat City yourself.

THE DIET BORE

Former fatties who have lost weight and cannot stop talking about it. All their pals know every morsel they've eaten that day, what the scale said, what they're going to cheat eat on their Controlled Cheating Days, and on which days they can cheat.

When asked how they did it, they go on and on until people get ill or someone finally says, "I'm sorry I asked." Every dinner conversation is sprinkled with long lists of what they can and cannot eat.

Diet Bores always talk in a loud enough voice to take a blue ribbon at an Ozark hog-calling contest. Well, it takes one to know one, as they say. And hogging conversation with your diet talk is as unappetizing as hogging food (the way you did—but you don't do anymore).

DIET MARTYR

A hot-stuff dieter on a Non-Cheating Day who sits down to eat with someone else—with family, at a banquet, etc.—and sadly and silently suffers with eyes cast down at broiled fish and salad with fresh lemon dressing. The weight of the eating world is on his back and his chin is resting on the table. O pity me!

DIET WATCHER

A tasteless Goal Weighter who stares at other people's food while they are eating. Each bite, taste, slurp, and crumb is recorded on the eyeballs lovingly and longingly by the Diet Watcher. This is the most dangerous of all Diet Don'ts. You could end up with a plate of hot lasagna in the face.

Take heed of these little tips. Years ago I saw the eyes of friends glaze over with boredom and anger with my self-righteous nincompoopery. I'm lucky to have a chubby pal left.

THIS IS
WAR!!!

The Battlefield: Any restaurant or beanery, holiday, outdoor barbecue, pal's dinner party, relative's roundup, picnic, soiree, wedding, or mob scene of more than two but less than twenty thousand people where there is the ENEMY: the dreaded Army of Fattening Foods on a Non-Cheating Day.

The Soldier: You, Controlled Cheater. Women and men are both drafted in this person's army. Both have to be on the front lines ready to do battle with the ENEMY.

The Offense: The ENEMY generals are the hostess and host wanting to smite you with their swords of warm Italian garlic bread and butter.

The Defense: You. YOU trying to diet in full battle uniform.

THE BATTLE UNIFORM

Helmet: To protect you from the rain of salty cashews that the ENEMY keeps firing at you from cute little dishes on every coffee table.

Battle Jacket: A trim-fitting Levi denim jacket with pockets to hold your ammunition: .32 caliber cantaloupe and raw carrot mortars.

Battle Belt: Metal rings from the tops of diet soda cans linked together to hold your low-calorie canteen filled with A & W Sugar-free Root Beer. Also five rings to attach your Red Delicious apple grenades. The Battle Belt also holds up your pants, which have become too big from winning all those pitched battles with the ENEMY.

Combat Boots: Special Nike Diet Running Shoes made for Controlled Cheaters. The soles are heavy sponge romaine lettuce leaves for twisting and turning quickly to avoid the most powerful weapon of the ENEMY: The "Goody Table" Tank.

Your Weaponry: YOUR MOUTH. The devastating, thirty-two-tooth, Mint Crest-brushed arsenal. The most powerful Controlled Cheating weapon in the world shoots only three bullets: NO THANK YOU.

Your mouth is your automatic rifle. It is easy to carry and can deliver a defensive punch that has never failed to make the ENEMY retreat to their foxholes and the garbage disposals.

When offered a plate of pepperoni pizza, turn your rifle and shoot oh-so-politely, NO THANK YOU. You will never run out of bullets.

THE ENEMY WEAPON

The "Goody Table" Tank: An awesome ENEMY war machine that has laid low many a Controlled Cheater. This brutal baby has some of the most powerful guns in the battle. The Tank fires plates of cheese, cakes, cookies, quiche, and corn bread; bowls of sour-cream dip, potato chips, pretzels, peanuts, and M&M's.

The vicious "Goody Table" Tank has a secret weapon, too. A human magnet that draws heat-seeking Controlled Cheating bodies to it. These poor bodies many times have no control once within the reach of the dreaded Goody Table.

Never you fret. You are lucky to have that rough-and-ready winner of the Congressional Medal of Slimness, Controlled Cheating combat veteran, ruggedly good-looking with just a touch of gray at the temples, Commander in Chief of All Allied Forces in the Bakery Department of Safeway, honors graduate of the Dairy Queen Military Academy, and all-around, Baby Ruth chewing, tough son-of-a-gun dieter "Ike, Omar, Patton, Dutch" Goldberg as your commander.

The following are General Goldberg's famous defensive strategies that have been carefully studied by every ENEMY party-giver from here to Arkansas:

The Famous Kitchen Slide: Dieter steps into a Christmas Day dinner, wedding reception, birthday party, or any other battle and stumbles unsuspecting on the ENEMY'S favorite battleground. The kitchen.

Quickly move your Combat Boots and slide sideways through the crowd and move directly into the bedroom. Start looking for what your enemy has in the drawers of their night table. Never, *never* do battle in the kitchen. You're always outnumbered.

Mata Hari and Mata Harry: These tricksters are your host and hostess, under heavy disguise to lure you into a dangerous high-calorie eating trap.

Some of their favorite ploys are hiding brownies under your salad, cherry pie disguised as broccoli, and luscious, greasy fried chicken molded in the shape of plain yogurt. Beware!

Hitting the Beach at Coney Island on D-Day: Soldier, make sure you have your Rifle, Helmet, Battle Jacket, Battle Belt, and Combat Boots when you invade any picnic, barbecue, beach cookout, or other battle fought out-of-doors in the fresh air without cover.

The ENEMY knows that everything tastes better outdoors, what with homemade potato salad, juicy hot barbecued hamburgers and hot dogs, corn on the cob drenched in two sticks of butter, all washed down with cold beer and soda. For dessert there's your aunt's chocolate cake with gooey, creamy frosting that you have to lick off your hands.

When you hit the beach, dig in and have only one burger well done, plenty of diet soda, and two bushels of fresh fruit including all the watermelon you can handle.

When the ENEMY sees this, they will turn tail and retreat. You've defeated them again.

Nerve Gas: The sneakiest, dirtiest trick in the ENEMY'S arsenal, nerve gas cannot be seen, smelled, or heard. Horribly, it can attack at any large or small party, where you don't know a soul and you're trying to find someone to talk to.

Or it can creep up at an Easter Sunday dinner where the Easter Bunny just laid an egg.

Or when you're invited to a married couple's small intimate dinner party and they've invited someone "who is just perfect for you."

You guessed it. Nerve gas causes nerves and nervousness, the silent enemy. Twitching hands go into key lime pies, and mouths suddenly can open wide enough to accommodate a whole pan of lasagna.

When you're chatting with someone truly wonderful, and you're draped against the bookcase to look as skinny as possible, and the light, witty conversation suddenly drops dead, and your mind turns to oatmeal, I guarantee the awful nerve gas will attack.

Your only counterattack is to muster your mighty DIET. Call up your secret reserves: RESOLVE AND NERVE.

Drop your hands to your sides and let them dangle. Do not raise them higher than your knees. Square your shoulders and jaw and see if you've got any carrot mortars or apple grenades left. If not, ask the wonderful person to go out on the terrace to watch the submarine races, or into the hall to play with the elevator buttons, or escort them in to see the new shower curtain.

Whatever you do, Soldier, walk, sprint, or run as fast and far as possible from the ENEMY. Get internally tough and think about your Controlled Cheating Day coming up.

Now a word from the Commander in Chief:
"Troops, you will never see V.E. Day, Victory over Eating. You will never get a ticker-tape parade down Broadway when you return from the Diet Wars. You will never be total victors.

"You will be doing battle with the ENEMY for the rest of your born days. You will have furloughs on your Controlled Cheating Days, but you will never experience complete victory over fattening foods.

"Take it from this old diet soldier, you will have to fight, gouge, and kick the ENEMY whenever this foul thing rears its ugly head on Non-Cheating Days.

"By now, you are wise, battle-hardened veterans, who can beat back any food challenge.

"Remember, old dieters never die, they just melt away."

HOW TO EAT DELICIOUS AND NUTRITIOUS FOODS WHILE GOING OUT, ORDERING IN, FACING FAST FOODS, SHOVING SLOW FOODS, APPROACHING STRANGE FOREIGN FOODS, AT PALS' PARTIES, ENEMIES' PARTIES, BROWN BAGGING, PICNICS, AND RAIDING OTHER FOLKS' REFRIGERATORS.

This is a smorgasbord of tips I've used, invented, heard from pals, read about, and learned from my sky writers. All these Controlled Cheating bumper stickers are dumped and mixed up like a good pizza pie. Each one will be new and fresh.

- The big news is that you eat *away* from the house exactly the way you eat *in* the house.
- The laws for healthy eating are the same wherever you put on the feed bag. This means wherever you eat you remember

your Controlled Cheating diet foods and select exactly the same foods as on any other Diet Day.

- Before you start Controlled Cheating, GO SEE YOUR DOCTOR!
- Pizza and popsicles in Hollywood, California, have the same fat and calories as they do in your kitchen.
- Eat foods that are broiled, roasted, steamed, poached, baked, or stir-fried with a little oil.
- Watch out for fried, french-fried, breaded, buttered, creamed, hollandaised, scalloped, au gratin, pickled, smoked, marinated, crispy, and braised.
- Study all menus as though you're decoding a secret message from the CIA.
- Become a taster, not a shoveler. The fifth bite of an apple pie has the same flavor as the first. Take *one* bite at a time.
- Exercise! Move that tush.
- For all Diet Days, follow the "Take My Diet, Please" chapter. You're already a diet professional.
- Talk a lot when you're eating. You may not be invited back, but who cares, you'll be skinny.
- Don't you dare pick up that salt shaker.
- If you want a walnut brownie or any other goody on a Diet Day, wait fifteen minutes . . . then imagine you've thrown it out the window.
- Leave food on the plate. I have a real problem with this one. I pour salt, pepper, and water all over the stuff that is still on the plate.
- Order à la carte. Skip the blue plate special

with five courses, especially if they are covered in gravy.

- Hooray, more restaurants are serving low-fat, low-calorie foods now. See if your pals know any eateries that have "spa" food.
- No cholesterol doesn't mean fat free.
- Slow down. The food will still be there.
- Get up now and take a twenty-minute walk.
- You don't have to order dessert.
- Eat "fresh" as much as possible.
- Always use small plates. Smaller portions will look larger.
- Trim all visible fat from meat. Use a sharp sword.
- Portions are huge at restaurants. Order an extra plate and split with someone else. Saves money too, and you get more flavors.
- You can order lobster (big bucks), but you get no butter.
- Drink two glasses of water NOW!
- Order foods that require work, like cutting, gnawing, picking, sucking, and plenty of horsing around. A good piece of bony chicken or turkey can take forty-five minutes to eat. You'll eat less and make lots of noise.
- When ordering, know exactly what you want and do not change, regardless of what the others order. Take no guff from the server.
- Eat fresh fruit, if anything, for dessert.
- Don't yo-yo up and down.
- Stay away from cold cuts, luncheon meats, and cheese. They have many hidden calories and fat.
- Take the skin off turkey and chicken. This is where the fat hides. You'll save a lot of calories.

- If you've got food left on your plate, ask for a Goldberg Bag and take the rest home for another meal.
- Pick at your food.
- Use your imagination. It's the most important and powerful diet muscle we have.
- Forget duck and goose. Very, very fatty fowl. Heavy calories.
- See your doctor before going on this diet.
- Order your pizza with whole wheat crust, if available, half the low-fat cheese, or no cheese, and all the vegetables they can heap on.
- Love those baked potatoes. Add a little margarine, low-fat cottage cheese, lemon or lime juice, chives, onions, low-fat yogurt, a little drizzle of olive oil, beans, and other veggies.

OR

"Attention ladies and gentlemen, now substituting for sour cream . . ." Here are two great recipes.

Blend equal parts low-fat cottage cheese and low-fat yogurt.

Blend one cup low-fat cottage cheese, two tablespoons low-fat buttermilk, and two teaspoons fresh lemon juice.

(A tablespoon of fat has 120 calories.)

- Olive and canola are better than other vegetable oils—more monosaturated fat.
- Eat small meals frequently . . . like a bird, not a vulture.
- Bagels don't have any fat. But don't eat egg bagels. Most French breads don't have any fat either.
- Call the eatery you're going to and find out what's on the menu and how it's prepared.

Even better, schlep over and get the poop in person.
- Use YOUR POWER.
- Choose two or three appetizers instead of the main course.
- Stuffed? Take a walk.
- Not stuffed? Take a walk.
- Share with a friend, unless he has a bigger fork than you.
- LOVE YOUR BODY. Hug yourself. It's the only one you've got.

THE BROWN BAG LUNCH

Brown Bagging:
- Saves time
- Saves calories and fat
- Saves money
- You control what you stuff in that bag.
- Eat a variety of foods like you've been doing; low-fat, high-fiber foods such as fresh fruits, vegetables, whole grains, poultry, and lean meat.
- Watch out for processed luncheon meats. They could be loaded with fat and salt. Read those labels.
- Spend a few bucks for a Thermos jug or insulated box to keep your food hot and cold.
- Watch out for drinks and desserts at lunchtime. These babies could be loaded with fat and sugar.
- Psst. I'll bet you two cheeseburgers that most "brown baggers" have peanut butter and jelly sandwiches in their bag. That's my all time favorite too. Try slicing fresh

bananas, apples, or pears on the peanut butter instead of jelly.

- Sandwich safety:
  1. Carry chilled foods in an insulated bag or box.
  2. Freeze your sandwich. By lunch time, it will be thawed.
  3. Put your sandwich in a refrigerator until lunchtime. Fillings made with meat, fish, or eggs can spoil if kept at room temperature for more than two hours. That includes sandwiches made with mayonnaise, mayonnaise-type dressing, or hard-cooked eggs. Seventy percent of Brown Baggers are adults. Some even carry Ninja Turtle lunch boxes.
- Now that you've got all that extra time gained by bringing your lunch, take a fast walk.
- When you go to work you'll look great sporting a brown bag in your Brooks Brothers suit or Liz Claiborne dress.

FIGHTING BOREDOM

Boredom in any eatery is dangerous for us. You can't run away; you can't start reading *Mad* magazine; you have to sit there where your idle little hands can pick up little french fries from someone else's plate and slide them into your rosebud mouth, which then won't be idle.

My favorite cure for boredom, when I'm not having a good time, is to take a peaceful cruise into my imagination. I dream about me and Barbra Streisand starring in *The Weight We Were*. Or better yet, I daydream about what I'm going to eat on my next Controlled Cheating Day.

ANOTHER BARRAGE OF TIPS
FOR THE BATTLEFIELD

- Fresh strawberries and other fruits are a dynamite low-calorie dessert. No sour cream either, sneaky.
- The three best, most important words for a dieter, are NO THANK YOU. Maybe you should ink those ten letters on your knuckles.
- Order NO complete meals. Get everything separately—as they say in France, à la carte.
- The big advantage in Chinese restaurants is that almost everything is cooked to order. So you can get anything you want cooked the way you want it—no salt, oil, or MSG.
- Don't eat foods you don't like.
- Malcolm Forbes said, "Dessert is my favorite vegetable."
- One gimmick I used for years when I was fat was to help the hostess or host clear the table. I could knock off 5,000 more calories in the kitchen eating mashed potatoes and gravy with my fingers. You just sit there and be rude—and thin.
- Be sure you eat tiny bites of everything. No shoveling.
- Have the waitress bring salad dressings and all sauces on the side, if you want a little taste. Then you can control how much is sprayed on.
- As best you can, keep an empty refrigerator. Only keep what you absolutely must

have for your family. I live alone. My fridge looks like I'm ready to move to Moscow.

- Half of the meals we eat are outside the house. Better learn how to order and nosh in a restaurant.
- On Diet Days, cut out the three whites—salt, sugar, and bleached flour.
- Talking, when you're out eating, has fewer calories than french-fried potatoes.
- At a big party, where no one is watching, you can diet to your heart's content. Watch out, you can cheat to your heart's content, too.
- Look in your mirror. Be honest.
- Never go back for "seconds."
- If it's a Diet Day and you're at a friend's house for dinner, so they won't get upset because you're not eating enough, give them loads of compliments and smack your lips a lot.
- Cut your food into small pieces.
- Drink a glass of water as soon as you sit down at the table.
- Don't pick food off other folks' plates. It's rude unless it's your mother's plate.
- Never give up.
- At a party, stay as far away as possible from the goody table without ending up on the front lawn or in the tree house.
- YOU pick and choose.
- On Controlled Cheating Days, don't waste calories on dumb cheating foods you don't really want. Become a class junk-food eater.
- Have four belly laughs and three hugs every day.
- Plan your whole eating day when you know you're going out.

- You order first. Don't listen to the other folks. Stick to your eating guns.
- At a party, stay out of the kitchen and forty-three miles from the table of eats.
- You don't have to eat everything on the plate. Mush the food around.
- Grab a sweetie pie and dance your tootsies off at a party. Great exercise and you keep busy. Also mingle. You might find the person of your dreams.
- Order a diet soda pop or seltzer when you get to the café or party. These will give you gas and fill you up.
- Try something new from the café menu. Open up. Be flexible. Be an explorer like Lawrence of Arugula. Look at the *whole* menu.
- Use your imagination. Don't eat the "same old thing" all the time. Loosen up.
- Going out to a seafood restaurant? Order the fish poached, baked, broiled, boiled, or grilled on a dry grill. Hold the butter and tartar sauce. Hit that fish with plenty of fresh lime or lemon juice.
- Eat half of the goodies on your plate if the portions are big enough for a giraffe.
- Try a health food or vegetarian eatery. Stay away from the nuts and seeds—too many calories and fat. Wear a tie-dyed T-shirt and a long-haired wig with a pony tail.
- When you eat very slooooowly, the taste of the food comes through like a freight train.
- The twenty potato chips you slip in your mouth at a party will cost you as many calories as you would spend in two hours normally sitting and shuffling cards.
- Remember, you're not a kid anymore.

You, Controlled Cheater, don't have to join the "Clean Plate Club"!

- Always order diet soda, low-sodium tomato juice, or one of the fancy waters with a spritz of lime. Only order the fancy water when you're not paying.
- Take a multivitamin and mineral supplement every day.
- Don't pick up your fork until everyone else has begun to eat.
- Forget cream sauces, butter sauces, or any sauces through which you can't see the bottom of the bowl.
- The roll basket is there for everyone. Don't become a "Diet Bore" by asking the server to take it away. You, Controlled Cheater, are not the only one at the table.

STAND UP BEFORE YOU SIT DOWN.

- No-fat doesn't mean low calorie.
- What fruit has the most fiber? Prunes. Get ready.
- Never announce you're on a diet. They'll find out soon enough when they see your slim body.
- Mess around with the food on your plate to make it look like you've attacked the food. No sneaky tastes either, when they put on something fattening.
- Eat carrots, celery, cauliflower, or fruit, and drink a glass of water at your house before leaving for dinner at a friend's or a restaurant. Never go out when you're "starved."
- Ask for margarine on the side instead of butter.
- A big passionate kiss burns twelve calories. Umm-Umm.

- Get margarine, sauces, and all condiments "on the side."
- Send food back if it isn't fixed the way you ordered it. Don't be a scared chicken. Raise your feathers.
- Only eat what you love.
- Eat noisy, crunchy foods, like apples, broccoli, or carrots. The sounds will thrill your tummy and you'll think you're eating cashew nuts.
- Like cafeterias? I do. No complete meals to tempt us. Inspect the whole line before you grab your tray. Desserts are usually first. Be careful.
- Be sure everything isn't drenched in butter, grease, or salt.
- A potato has more vitamin C than an orange.
- A banana has more potassium than a potato.
- Calories, fat, and sodium can add up quicker than a man with three hands in a smorgasbord. If you order a quarter pound hamburger, large size fries, and a vanilla shake, you consume 1,205 calories, 59 grams of fat, and 1,655 milligrams of sodium. Hold off until your Cheating Day.
- Smear your margarine on cool bread. If the bread is hot, it will soak in the bread and you'll use more. It's a visual thing.
- Become a taster instead of an eater at parties, beaneries, and friends' houses.
- Finally, one of the best pieces of diet advice I ever got: (This one is so hard to do I've been working on it for twenty-four years with just a little success. You do it too, because it's worth the effort.)

PUT YOUR FORK OR SPOON DOWN AFTER EVERY BITE. DO NOT PICK IT UP UNTIL AFTER YOU HAVE CHEWED THE FOOD SLOOOOOWLY AND SWALLOWED.

You'll be amazed at how slowly you'll eat, how much more you'll enjoy your goodies, how much less you'll eat, and how quickly you'll get full.

VACATION
CHEATING

C.H.E.A.T.,
The Congress of Healthy Eating
All the Time,

NEW UNION CONTRACT CONCERNING
VACATIONS, CHEATING, AND NON-CHEATING

The Union Meeting to be held on The Good Ship Lollipop.

"Attention. May I have your attention, please. Will the members tear themselves away from the salad bar and please find seats. There are plenty of good seats in the front. I won't bite you, unless I get really hungry.

"First, the membership committee would like to welcome the new members, the Goal Weighters, who have served their diet apprenticeship and are now entitled to all benefits and privileges accorded the membership of the beloved C.H.E.A.T. Union.

"As your president, Cuisine Art, I must tell you that we have had some problems in the Bread Board Room during the negotiations with the executive board and certain shop stewards.

"I hate to report to the membership that Sara Lee punched out the Pillsbury Dough Boy. Chef Boyardee resigned as vice president in charge of ravioli. Popeye chickened out on marrying Ann Page, who promptly hit him in the face with one of her pumpkin pies. Ronald McDonald and the Burger King are still not speaking, due to both being in love with Wendy. Colonel Sanders stormed out in a huff when we ordered in fried chicken from Brown's. Other than these insignificant problems, everything went as smooth as Dannon Lemon Yogurt.

"There is one sad announcement. Irving Shakey of Shakey's Pizza is retiring from active membership. He and the missus will be retiring to Hershey, Pennsylvania, where they will try to invent a chocolate anchovy. Irving wanted me to tell all of you he'd sure be pleased if you'd stop by and see them in Hershey. The missus said they'd always have a bed for you in an abandoned pizza oven.

"Irving, as one of our charter members, we're going to miss you.

"On to the terms of the Vacations Contract with Fats Goldberg and his Controlled Cheating Corporation. We have done some hard, heavy bargaining that went nonstop for six and a half months. The executive committee, the shop stewards (when they weren't fighting), and I have come up with what we think is a fair agreement with Fats Goldberg concerning our rights to eat on vacations.

"Will the sergeant at arms, Dairy Queen,

please pass out copies of the new Vacation Contract. There is one negative note. Due to recession there will be a Tastee Freeze on wages."

VACATIONS: THE C.H.E.A.T. UNION CONTRACT

(To be posted at all water fountains, soda and candy machines, and anywhere that calories are dispensed.)

Article One: *You may Controlled Cheat every other day on your vacation.*

Rejoice and celebrate. Applaud yourself. Your new contract really says you can have every other day a Controlled Cheating Day!

VACATION!

Every morning, your happy eyes open like pistachio nuts and stare at the candy-striped pillow case. A big grin sweeps across your face, getting a mouthful of candy-striped lint. You wake up to either plan your Controlled Cheating Day or to fondly remember the one you just had, and plan for tomorrow.

It makes no difference whether you're sleeping under the stars in your camper in West Texas, under silk sheets in The Carlyle Hotel in New York City, under a blinking no-vacancy sign at a Ramada Inn in Santa Barbara, California, or under your own roof in Arlington Heights, Illinois; you, Controlled Cheater, are on vacation.

What a combination. A well-deserved rest from work and a well-served Cheating Eating Vacation. The best two (nonconsecutive) weeks of your year!

This is some big eating deal for you. But, like all good union contracts, there are certain key provisions that *must* be followed to stay in compliance with Fats Goldberg and the Controlled Cheating Corporation.

You are a valued member of the organization and we would be totally lost without you. Your diet productivity and personality are essential to the success of the company. Besides, you bake dynamite walnut brownies. You are indispensable. We need you back, so please read the rules and regulations carefully for your Cheating Eating Vacations.

Provision: *Goal Weight.* No Controlled Cheater may go on an every-other-day Cheating Vacation until they have been at Goal Weight for AT LEAST THREE MONTHS.

You know as well as I do why that rule is in the contract. I want you to be completely comfortable in your new Goal Weight life. So content and easy with Controlled Cheating that you'll be able to go back on your diet as easily as you would slip on your favorite maroon felt carpet slippers.

Three or four days of good time eating is one heck of a lot of goodies. You're a professional Controlled Cheater after all these months. Being the boss eater, I have confidence in your reliability. You will return to the Cheating Eating assembly line with renewed vigor and snapshots of the meals you ate.

Provision: *You May Not Cheat Two Weeks in a Row on Your Vacation.* Let's go over that again. You may NOT, under any silly circumstances, for any reasons, excuses, or alibis whatever, vacation cheat for two straight weeks. Talk about blowing your whole diet. This would be it. Taking a two-weeks-in-a-row eating vacation is as risky as going to dinner at a skinny couple's home where they serve Cheez Whiz on Ritz Crackers instead of a salad.

If I let you take fourteen days in a row of cheating every other day, you'd be sliding down that fat road faster than Al Unser cruises at the Indianapolis 500.

You've worked too hard to blow it all at once. I tried two straight weeks of eating every other day about fifteen years ago. It took everything I had to get back to my Goal Weight. I'll talk about that later.

Once more, for the delayed broadcast to the West Coast: You may not take your two-week Cheating Eating Vacation in one huge gulp. One week at a time is it.

Provision: *No Bozo Eating.* Look, you know all there is to know about bozo or crazy eating. You've educated yourself from your Controlled Cheating Days. We'll go over nutsy eating just once more because it's vitally important in your every-other-day-eating vacation: *Only eat when you're hungry and only eat foods you truly crave.*

Planning is as important for these Cheating Days as the cone is to ice cream. You're looking at three or four days of big time, high-level dining. That's ninety-six hours of fun twice a year.

Make sure you eat a whole variety of good foods. Go to places you didn't have time for on your regular Controlled Cheating Days. Nosh your way around town. Or have a barbecue at home. Do anything and everything you want in the eating department. Use your imagination: Don't fool around with no-fun, no-flavor washouts like white bread, American cheese, and miniature marshmallows.

Provision: *How to Cheat and Diet When You Are Gone for Two Weeks or Longer on Vacation.*

You must stick to your normal cheating twice a week the first week and cheat the second week, not the other way around. If you cheat the first week of your vacation and try to diet on the second, the Las Vegas odds on you are 1,000,000 to 1 that you won't stop cheating the second week.

It's going to be tougher than nickel steak for you not to cheat the first week of your vacation, even though you planned to diet that first week. But you must stick to it!

If you actually plan to cheat the first week of your vacation and diet the second, I'm standing here eyeball to eyeball telling you that you're going to cheat every other day for fourteen straight days. This will be a disaster and jeopardize your whole Controlled Cheating program.

Unless you always dreamed of being a kamikaze pilot in World War II, *do not do it!*

Provision: *How to Eat on Diet Days When You're on Vacation and Other Trips.* Surprise! You eat exactly the same way you do at home when you got out to eat.

Provision: *How to Exercise When You're on Vacation and Other Trips.* Surprise! You exercise and move that tush just like you do at the homestead. If you are flying, walk from one end of the airport to the other, instead of sitting and waiting for your plane. Plan your trip so you can sightsee on foot.

Provision: *Eating on the Run, or Controlled Cheat Dining in Public Transportation and Your Own Car.*

AIRPLANE EATING

Everyone laughs and makes fun of the food served on airplanes. It's good for a few giggles from your bored friends who always have hilarious airline food stories of their own. We've all had the beige Salisbury steaks, pink cake, and pitted peas on Flight 99 nonstop from Lima to Columbus, Ohio.

The good news is that most airlines offer us serious Controlled Cheaters a big selection of low-calorie and special meals along with their astronomical fares.

You must ask for a special meal at least twenty-four hours in advance or preferably when you make your reservation. Here are just a few of the dietetic and special meals you can order:

- Low-calorie or diabetic
- Cold seafood platter (my favorite)
- Vegetarian
- Low-sodium or salt-free
- Fruit plate
- Low cholesterol
- Kosher

Beware those high-fat, high-calorie nibbles. Say "no thanks" and play with the light switch and air control.

SHIPS, TRAINS, AND BUSES

Ships: The only large, floating object that I've been to sea with was my old 325-pound body. The biggest boat I've ever been on was the Circle Line Cruise boat around the island of Manhattan where they serve terrible hot dogs and great frozen custard.

What I hear from folks who go on grown-up cruises for their vacations is that a ship is a dieter's nightmare. It's nonstop feeding from early morning until late at night with snacks in between.

Sorry, you're going to have to tooth-check ships yourself. Be very, very careful.

Trains and buses: Bring a Sears shopping bag with your own goodies.

CAR CUISINE

The automobile and I have had an eating love affair for all my born days. There have been seven beautiful cars in my past. The first was sold to me by two of my uncles, Jimmy and Harry, who owned A-to-Z Auto Wrecking. They pulled a 1937 Oldsmobile from the pile and gave it to me for $30. It was love at first sight. But my baby had a problem. Every time I stopped, all the oil in the motor leaked out on the ground. No one would let me park in their driveway. All my money went for food and oil.

I ate well in that car. Twice a week I had to sweep the floors in both front and back because the build-up of watermelon seeds, Dolly Madison cake wrappers, caramel corn, and crumbs from cheeseburgers made it unbecoming.

In 1960 I bought a brand new Volkswagen Beetle (which I sold in 1965 when I moved from Chicago to New York). That baby was an insurance policy for me after I went from 325 pounds to 190 in 1959. The sun roof model with push-button radio and white walls cost $1,812 and was a great incentive to stay skinny. If I put on two pounds, I'd never be able to fit in the front seat again.

My eyes glaze over with tears of eating happiness when I think about all the delicious groceries I've devoured in the seats and on the running boards of those seven rolling lunch boxes.

Make sure you get a stick shift. It's almost impossible to eat and drive.

Give me a car and a highway and I start daydreaming of roadside burger joints, soft ice cream, and the one and only, best eating of them all, gas stations. Yeah, gas stations. They have a limited menu, the service is fast, and the food is cheap.

My love affair with dining in gas stations started when I was growing up on Thirty-ninth and Agnes in Kansas City. There were two gas stations across the street.

One was a Texaco station owned by the Meyers brothers. The candy machine had only a fair selection. It was heavy on packages of peanut butter spread on orange-colored crackers. The Coke machine was a treat and not only had Coke but Mission Orange and Mason's Root Beer.

The other station was a Phillips 66 owned by my cousin, Dave. The Coke machine was so-so, with only Coke, 7-Up, and Grapette. The candy machine was okay. What they did have was a one-cent peanut machine that gave you a handful of the saltiest, greasiest peanuts in the world.

I'm going to give you one of the only two recipes I know in the whole world. The first is for all kinds of pizzas.

This is the other one:
1. Take one ice-cold bottle or can of Coca-Cola.
2. Gulp down two large swigs.
3. Get the greasiest, saltiest peanuts you can buy, preferably with the red skins still on.
4. Take a medium handful of peanuts and pour them in the Coke. You can lick the palm of your hand for the extra salt.

5. Take a gurgle of Coke and peanuts and start chewing that heavenly mixture of Coke, peanuts, salt, and grease. You might never come back to earth.

Dieting in cars, campers, trailers, or anything else that rolls on highways or dirt roads is easy on vacations. You and the Dalton Gang in the back seat are a self-contained unit. No goodies can come in except those that you buy and put on the seat.

All those roadside eateries do reach out their yummy paws and want to drag you in. But you have the flexibility to roar on down that road.

When I used to have a car and drive and diet, I'd always have a big bag of fruit on the front seat next to me. I could reach in and whip out a peach, apple, plum, or anything else. My sticky steering wheel smelled like a fruit cocktail. Also take along small cans or cartons of juice, a jar of peanut butter, some whole wheat bread, and a snack mix of popcorn, unsweetened cereals, and bite size pretzels.

I always get the popcorn all over the floor. Take along one of those coolers to keep everything frigid.

There are also advantages in highway diet eating. You can stop at roadside farm stands and buy fresh-picked vegetables direct from the field that's twelve feet away. There's absolutely nothing better than a fresh-picked homegrown tomato that you eat like an apple.

When you stop for gas, stay in the car. Don't mosey around the station looking in the goody machines unless it's a Cheating Day.

Another advantage of dieting in an automobile is that gas prices are so high you won't have any extra money to eat anyway.

Provision: *You Must Leave Your Scale at Home.* Leave that baby on the bathroom floor. When I say vacation, I mean vacation from everything, including the tyranny and twitchiness of hopping on the scale every morning.

There are times I wanted to take my scale with me on vacations. I thought I'd buy a velvet-lined scale satchel from Samsonite for easy carrying. They haven't invented one yet. But I stifled the urge, kissed my Health-O-Meter good-bye, locked the door, and happily danced down the stairs, free at last.

Provision: *You Must Go Back on Your Diet After Vacation.* You are going to panic. I know, because I've panicked every six months for the last thirty-two years. The panic attacks you the moment you open your eyes the morning after the Vacation Eating Week of Controlled Cheating.

Panic Button #1: This button pushes that part of your mind that says, "How in the world can I go back on that awful low-calorie balanced diet after I've had a fun-filled week of uninterrupted eating? I'm going to stay under these covers the rest of my life."

Off Button #1: You can turn Panic Button #1 off because you only have six short days of dieting before you can cheat again. That's *six days* of low-calorie balanced dieting. After those six days, you have your regular Cheating Eating Day. Then it's back to your twice-a-week program. Once more, that is *six days of dieting* be fore you can cheat again. Dream back over your Eating Vacation and relive those magic masticating moments.

All right, chorus, let's hear your old favorite hymn. First the sopranos, then the altos and basses, you come right in. Ready?

"I Must Go Back on My Diet." Sing that song again.

"I MUST GO BACK ON MY DIET." Solid!

Panic Button #2: After you crawl out of bed and after you turn off Panic Button #1, you must weigh yourself.

Yes, you must stand up straight, look dead ahead, and resolutely walk to where your scale is hiding. Without any fuss, climb up on your scale and look directly down at the dial. No hesitating.

Off Button #2: Before you step on the scale, turn on the shower, radio, and television full force. This will drown out your whimpers, cries, or screams without bothering the rest of the family.

After you've gotten that out of your system, you'll be fine. Who cares what that dumb dial says? You had a great seven days. You planned it all out, so there is no guilt or depression. You knew exactly what you were doing every step of the way. And there are only six small days until you can Control Cheat again.

Don't expect the scale dial to go right back to your Goal Weight (the weight you were before you went on vacation) in six days. That is going to take time. But over a period of weeks your weight will gradually return to your Goal Weight. Above all, don't skip any Cheating Days. You still need them.

You'll probably even be glad to get back on your diet, because you feel so much better when you're lighter.

I sure wish there was some other way to do this, but . . . after you get back from Controlled Cheating Eating Vacation,

YOU MUST GO BACK ON YOUR DIET!

YOU MUST GO BACK ON YOUR DIET FOR SIX STRAIGHT DAYS! THEN YOU MAY HAVE A CHEATING EATING DAY. AFTER THAT IT IS BACK TO YOUR TWICE-A-WEEK CHEATING PROGRAM.

"I think we have a terrific contract here. Let's vote. Everybody in favor, yell *chocolate*. Everybody opposed, yell *celery*.

"Since no one yelled celery and the scream for chocolate was shattering, the new contract passes unanimously.

"Meeting adjourned."

COME BACK, LITTLE CHEATER

A SPECIAL MESSAGE FROM YOUR OLD PAL FATS GOLDBERG

You tried this diet for six days and you were wonderful with low-calorie balanced dieting. Then came your first Controlled Cheating Day. You loved it so much you never went back to the diet part. Now it's six months later and you can't understand why you haven't lost a pound.

Or, one month, six months, one year, or six years from now the same thing happens. You hit a Controlled Cheating Day and you can't stop. You are on that diet roller coaster again going straight up.

Although Controlled Cheating works well for most people, sometimes you can't help yourself and you fall off the wagon. You can start again. We accept repeater cheaters, fallen angels, and other sugar-coated sinners. It's very easy to climb back on board in one simple step: JUST GO BACK TO PAGE ONE AND START ALL OVER AGAIN! I still like you.

DON'T GIVE UP YOUR DAY JOB

A good year—1961. I was dancing along in Chicago dieting and fairly happy. The dieting was tough as the bark on a tree, or easy as pie, or somewhere in between, depending on what day it was.

Over a long period of time, a revolutionary idea started in my toes and worked its way up to my Pepsi-soaked brain. *Dieting is like a job. A full-time job. Your second job.* The more I thought about it the truer it became. Losing weight and keeping it off is exactly like a job. Each morning I had to get up to go to not one, but two jobs.

One job was to slip on an oxford-cloth shirt, rep tie, over-the-calf socks, a Brooks Brothers suit, and Florsheim Imperial plain-toed cordovans and go to work at the *Chicago Tribune.* The other was getting up every morning and going to my job of dieting. Both were equally important. One job gave me enough loot to put doughnuts on the table. The other job was not to eat them (except on Controlled Cheating Days).

Don't give up your regular job when you take on the additional task of dieting. Work at both. Don't worry. Moonlighting becomes you, especially as you get slimmer and slimmer!

Losing weight and keeping it off is waking each day to the job of taking care of your body. It's the same as getting up and taking care of the house and children, or going to the plant, office, store, truck, or construction site.

The successful Controlled Cheating program is a full-time job, the same as any other job but with some big differences.

1. Keeping slim is a twenty-four-hour-a-day duty, not an eight-hour deal with time and a half for overtime and a break every three hours. We don't get paid with more food for working overtime on a diet.
2. There are no foremen, bosses, or other honchos to keep an eye on what you're doing and tell and show you what to do. You're totally in business for yourself!

When I noodled out that Controlled Cheating was a job, I also figured this was one of the main reasons why I, like most other fatties, couldn't lose weight and keep it off. We were looking at the problem in the wrong way.

All the time we'd think we could go on a diet for a while, maybe lose all the weight we wanted, and then relax and never put it on again. That's dead wrong.

At our jobs where we get paid, we don't work hard for a while and then relax and expect to get paid for the rest of our lives. If we did that, we wouldn't have the job. Why should dieting be any different? We have to get up every morning and "Go to dieting," like any job. Holding down two jobs is mean stuff. It takes hard work and everything we've got.

Hold on. Since dieting is like some tough job, how 'bout we get some of the benefits and goodies straight jobs have? We do. We do.

With Controlled Cheating in 1961, I had a day off, like my money job. As you know by now, after achieving Goal Weight, we have two days off, which is even better.

Again in 1961, I said, what about a vacation? Why not try? When I went to Kansas City on vacation, and had to diet, I was miserable. I thought, let me cheat every other day for a week and see if I can shake those pounds when I get back.

In the spring of 1962, I drove to Kansas City in my 1956 Chevy. Laughing all the way down Route 66, Highways 36, 54, and 40, I ate and vacationed for a week. In seven days, I put on seven pounds. It was staggering, but boy, did I have a supersensational vacation.

Sure, when I came back, I had to start dieting again. Who cared? With my Cheating Eating Vacation behind me, I could come back and go on my diet again, and I knew I was home free when it came to staying skinny the rest of my life.

Three weeks later I had lost the seven pounds. You've got to remember that I started my Controlled Cheating again immediately after six days of dieting.

That was nineteen years ago, and I still take a Cheating Eating Vacation twice a year. This job works for me and will work for you, too.

Some final points:

1. You can never retire from your diet job as you can from your straight job. No gold watch, no social security, no good-bye party. There is no job security either. You can never be secure when dieting. But you'll live a long and happy life.
2. You'll never get a raise, especially in pounds. Thank God!

So when you fall off your diet, consider it like losing a job. Sure, you're discouraged, but that doesn't mean you're going to spend the rest of your life on unemployment. Get back to work! Start back on the Controlled Cheating program, and remember, yesterday is ancient history.

COME BACK, LITTLE CHEATER. YOU CAN DO IT!

OVERWEIGHT KIDS AND CONTROLLED CHEATING

Shoot, if there had been a weight loss and maintenance program like Controlled Cheating when I was a kid, I wouldn't have blown up like the Goodyear Blimp floating over Kansas City.

I grew up in the Stone Age of losing weight and keeping it off. All the diets led nowhere. Those diets could kill you: a high-protein diet with lots of fatty meat; a carbohydrates-only diet; crunch rabbit food until you couldn't look at another lettuce leaf; and God forbid you should exercise. One of the biggest selling diet books in the 1950s warned: Never exercise because it will make you hungry and you'll only burn a few calories.

Looking back is dumb. Sure there were some tough spots along the way to me becoming a Jewish Adonis. Luckily, I got through childhood with a scratch, not a scar.

I guarantee that most overweight kids

will go crazy for Controlled Cheating. All the
good stuff that works for adults in Controlled
Cheating can work for children and adoles-
cents. Controlled Cheating has:

1. Healthy, nutritious, balanced eating
   that includes all the food groups with
   no calorie counting.
2. Exercise, Exercise, EXERCISE!
3. The Cheating Day.

A loving family is the best support system for a successful weight control program.
The family can make it a team effort, with a
cheering section; health can be a party. Enthusiastic, caring parents can help their children
avoid a lifetime of pain.

There's bad news from the fat wars:

- Twenty percent of the children in the
  U.S. are overweight.
- If the parents are obese, there's an 80
  percent chance the kids will be overweight.
- Obese ten- to thirteen-year-olds have a
  70 percent to 80 percent chance of being obese adults.
- The American Academy of Pediatrics
  warns that the single most important
  health problem today is overweight
  children.

Learning how to eat right is a family affair. Getting a good nutritional education is as
important as learning to read.

TIPS FOR OVERWEIGHT CHILDREN

- Schedule regular family meal times.
  With more parents working full time,

fewer families eat together. Hello, fast foods, goodbye nutrition.

- Forget counting calories—serve smaller portions and talk more during the meals.
- Parents should become beautiful models of good eating habits and exercise.
- Food should never be used as a prize or bribe. Give kids lots of positive reinforcement and a big hug.
- Throwing out all the foods with grease, dough, and sugar will not work. Like me, your children will go next door, to a bakery, or beg a frozen Snickers from a bus driver. Kids have to learn to handle all kinds of food, the earlier the better. Out of sight is *not* out of mind.

THE TELEVISION SET

Okay, pardner, it's prime time to zap the dirty, low-down varmint, the television. That sneaky villain has grabbed us with its slimy tentacles and sucked us into that dark hole. We've become dreaded couch potatoes. For myself, I'd rather be a french-fried couch potato, and I love television, too.

Experts say that kids are sitting and watching twenty-five hours of TV a week. Television has become an activity—or nonactivity.

Hold on. I'll bet a year's subscription to *TV Guide* that parents are watching that tube as much or more than their children. Don't blame everything on the kids. Nonstop television is a family problem.

What to do? What to do?

- Every adult should lift their big rear end off the chair, turn off the TV, and step out with the kids for a breezy walk, or take a bike ride, or wash the Rolls Royce, or dig for gold in the watermelon patch, or throw a Frisbee around, or roll around in the leaves with Shep, the dog. Move those gorgeous bodies. EXERCISE. Don't sit there.
- Have strict limits on how much and when your children can watch television.
- Get a stationary bike and have the family workout while watching the box. Have races on the stationary bike. Winner gets to sit in the recliner.
- Suggest they get involved in after-school activities like sports or acting class to cut down on television watching. Maybe the kids could get a part-time job making and baking pizzas. But make sure the job doesn't cut into their study time. Assign jobs around the house or no keys to the car.

Remember, parents, NO NAGGING. Better you should hug and kiss your overweight child. Then talk. The kid talks first. Then you talk. They talk. You talk. They talk. Both of you talk and hug.

Please, before your child or you go on Controlled Cheating, I ask you, with all my slim heart, go to your pediatrician or family doctor for a physical.

FAST, EASY, AND FEARLESS PIZZA

HOW TO MAKE AND EAT PIZZA AND LOSE WEIGHT

So how did a guy named Goldberg get into the pizza biz, with two Goldberg Pizzerias in New York City? The truth is . . . chicken soup made me sick.

People are passionate about pizza. I am passionate about pizza. There is nothing as satisfying as a delicious, gooey slice of pizza.

Pizza is almost the perfect, nutritious food, according to the Dietary Goals for the U.S., set by the Senate Select Committee on Nutrition and Human Needs.

The Slim Senators say that pizza has just the right percentages:

65% Complex Carbohydrates
20% Protein
15% Fat

Pizza is not a *junk* food.
More pizza is eaten in America than in

any other country in the whole world. Fourteen billion slices of pizza were sold last year. Bye, bye, burgers.

Pizza is a magic food. Basically, pizza is pure cheese, tomatoes, and dough. Darling, virginal pizza is the most versatile food in the whole history of eating. You can pile almost anything on top, animal, mineral, or vegetable, and still burn the roof of your mouth.

HOW TO MAKE A HEALTHY, NO-GUILT, HIGH-FIBER, LOW-FAT, LOW-SODIUM SLICE OF HEAVEN

GOLDBERG'S PIZZERIA TOMATO SAUCE

1 28 oz. can of whole tomatoes, preferably Italian, drained and hand crushed. Wash your hands first and watch out for squirts on your pants.
1 teaspoon basil
1 teaspoon oregano
1 tablespoon olive oil
Fresh garlic minced or chopped. I love lots of garlic. I'm leaving the amount up to you and your breath.

Directions: Now put all the ingredients in a bowl and mix until your arm gets tired. (No heating necessary.)

Remember: You cannot mess up a pizza. Have fun.

In a hurry to eat? Use a ready-made pizza or spaghetti sauce. They come in many flavors. (Check labels for fat, salt, and sugar.)

CRUSTS

Use Bagels, Pita bread, Italian bread, French bread, Flour tortillas, English muffins (the Wolferman's brand is best), sour dough bread, matzos, prebaked pizza crusts, or anything that will lay flat.

LOW FAT CHEESES

It is best to use part skim, low-moisture mozzarella, also called pizza cheese, or any skim or part-skim cheese.

Cheese substitutes have more fat and sodium than real cheese. Look for the word *substitute* on the label, then run away.

TOPPINGS

Select any kind of veggies and fruits— fresh of course. Add turkey, chicken (no skin), lean ground beef, veal, beans, water-packed tuna, shrimp, clams, mussels, scallops, lobster (if you can afford it), or any other fishy. Use your low-fat imagination. Almost anything works on a pizza.

INSTRUCTIONS FROM THE PIZZA PRINCE

HOW TO MAKE A PIZZA—GOLD-BERG STYLE. On top of the bagel, pita, or any other crust, spread one ounce of cheese. Add your toppings. Cover with another ounce of cheese. Add tomato sauce, a sprinkle of oregano and parmesan. Slip this beauty into your oven, toaster oven, microwave, or under the broiler. Remember, rare pizza is not so hot.

PIZZA POINTERS:
- Most low-fat cheeses are 80 calories an ounce.
- Pizza is cheap. Look in your ice box.

Use those low-fat, high-flavor leftovers.

- Watch out for two ingredients when
  making pizza: fat and salt. No pepperoni, sausage, or anchovies for you,
  buddy.
- Cut your toppings into small pieces
  and sprinkle all over. Then every bite
  is thrilling.
- Don't make a "blah" pizza. Use
  strong flavors for your toppings. Use
  fresh herbs if you can, and grind your
  black pepper.
- Try a "cheeseless" pizza.
- Frozen or delivered pizzas: Buy plain
  cheese pizza and add your own low-fat
  toppings, with extra spices and herbs.
  Remember, pepperoni is hell to peel
  off a hot pizza.
- Try dessert pizza with apples, cherries, peaches, or any other fresh fruits.
  If you do use canned fruits, make
  sure they're water packed.
- Pizza is a delicious waker-upper for
  breakfast. Don't pour milk on it.
- I once tried a chunky peanut butter
  and jelly pizza. Hot peanut butter and
  jelly looks like you know what and
  tastes the same.
- You can make your own pizza dough
  from scratch too. Bring the family.
  Make it a pizza party. Children love to
  make pizza. It's fun and sloppy. Or,
  stop by your local bakery and buy
  some bread dough. If you really and
  truly want to know how to make a
  pizzeria pizza from scratch, get *The*

Pizza Book by Evelyne Slomon. Or look in a dusty secondhand bookstore for *Goldberg's Pizza Book,* the first pizza cookbook in the world, written in 1971 by yours truly.

- Pizza is a beautiful, fragrant, and sensual extravaganza. I think I'll marry a garlic and onion pizza.
- Pizza is like sex: when its good it's terrific, and when it's bad, it's still pretty good.

Goldberg's Pizzerias have two famous pizzas you can make:

The SMOG Pizza: Sausage, Mushroom, Onion, and Green Peppers. This is the pizza that was named the Best Pizza in New York by *New York* magazine. You can substitute spinach for the sausage to make it low fat.

The Goldielox Pizza: Smoked Salmon and Onions. Try low-fat cream cheese with this one, bubbie.

There is only one rule for you to eat pizza on Diet Days: Eat *one* slice, or one bagel, or one pita bread *very sloooowwwly.* Don't eat a whole pizza unless it is four inches in diameter. Remember, MODERATION!

YOU ARE A SLIM STAR

Swami Goldberg says that it was written in the stars that pizza and losing weight can be enjoyed year-round. As the earth circles the sun and the planets shift their positions in the sky, making new horoscopes, the aspects are all favorable for pizza. I've been cogitating on different flavors of pizza for different zodiac signs, and have come to the conclusion that there may be something in the stars after all. I thought about baking one super zodiac pizza, with a slice for every sign, but difficulties stood in the way. First, it's tough to cut a pizza into twelfths. Second, the slices would be tiny—just a lick and a promise. And third, suppose there are two Capricorns in the crowd and no Cancers? You'd have to round up one person for each sign, which could be tough. Nowadays, you just can't go up to a stranger and say "What's your sign?" and not get clobbered. Plus certain signs don't get on too well with other signs, although love of pizza unites us all.

No, it's simpler to bake one pie for each sign. You can make a large pizza and invite only Libras, or you can make small individual pizzas and have a zodiac party. So, the chief astrologer at Goldberg's Pizzeria has come up with these well-aspected suggestions, all of them slim stars.

Aries the Ram: March 21–April 19

This fire sign is ruled by Mars, the red planet. Aries is characterized by action and fearlessness. Give the courageous ram a red pizza for the fearless eater. Mix fiery jalepeños in the tomato sauce. Spread on a garlic bagel; on top, garnish with strips of red pepper.

Taurus the Bull: April 20–May 20

Taurus is an earth sign, ruled by Venus. Steady, dependable, and not given to indigestion on Cheating Days. Taurus requires a sensuous pizza since his is the most sensuous sign of the twelve. Breathtaking garlic and noisy onions on a hunk of French bread are pretty sensuous, and besides, he can digest anything. (Ladies, NEVER eat this pizza alone with a Taurus.)

Gemini the Twins: May 21–June 20

This is an air sign ruled by Mercury, therefore the Gemini is mercurial and given to changes of mind. Try a combination of adorable black olives and lovely green olives on a whole wheat pita bread.

Cancer the Crab: June 21–July 22

A water sign ruled by the moon, Cancer is a home-loving sign, and the one most associated with food. Since Cancers adore elegance, their pizza should be beautiful, decorated, and colorful. Red and yellow onion rings with a little artistic artichoke make a pretty pattern for this sign. Then they won't get crabby.

Leo the Lion: July 23–August 22

A fire sign ruled by the sun, Leo is the most powerful and flamboyant sign in the zodiac—the lion is truly king of the jungle. Give him everything—the SMOG: spinach, mushrooms, onions, and green peppers. Make sure you pile on plenty, all the way down the lion.

Virgo the Virgin: August 23–September 22

Virgo is serious and precise, an earth sign whose ruling planet is Mercury. Pristine and critical, he'd better have the virginal cheese and tomato on a regular pizza crust with no fancy additions.

Libra the Scales:
September 23–October 22

An air sign ruled by Venus, Libra is intelligent, harmonious, and well balanced. Give them a broccoli bush and egg-citing eggplant on a perfect slice of sourdough bread.

Scorpio the Scorpion:
October 23–November 21

This erratic genius of the heavens is a water sign, ruled by both Pluto and Mars. This double protector gives Scorpios a fearless quality and an electric vitality; they are complex and fascinating. Spicy is the keynote for this pizza: spicy and vital. Lean ground beef with lots of spices and hot pepper flakes will take away the scorpion's sting.

Sagittarius the Archer:
November 22–December 21

The Sagittarian is generous, gregarious, and friendly, frank almost to the point of bluntness. Theirs is a fire sign ruled by Jupiter. For this open-minded and open-hearted sign, our astrologer suggests the frankest pizza there is: A heart-shaped pizza with turkey franks . . . an archer de triumph.

Capricorn the Goat:
December 22–January 19

A hard worker and industrious, the goat is ambitious and luxury loving, an earth sign ruled by Saturn. I'm a Capricorn. Boy, I didn't know I was that slick. The stars say that I like expensive pizza. Give me a shrimp, scallops, beans, and lots of fresh breathtaking garlic pizza on a pumpernickel bagel. Richard Nixon is a Capricorn, too. He probably puts ketchup on his pizza.

Aquarius the Water Bearer:
January 20–February 18

Born under an air sign ruled by Uranus, the Aquarian is warm natured and unpredictable. Try them on a moody mushroom pizza on Italian bread. Mushrooms like to wander all over the pizza when it's baking. As a famous Italian astrologer once said, "Pizza will come-a in our time."

Pisces the Fish: February 19–March 10

This last sign of the zodiac is a pure water sign, ruled by the king of the sea, Neptune. Pisceans tend to be lazy and living somewhere on Cloud Nine. They make up for it by being both charming and sexy. There's little choice here: fish all the way. A lobster pizza for sure, or clams, tuna, anchovies, and oysters. I'd like to take out a Pisces. As a famous Irish pizza astrologer once said, "This is the O'Fishal pizza for the Pisces."

MY
DIET
DAY

DIET DAYS, DEAR,
SWEET DIET DAYS

Struggling out of my sleepy diet rev-
eries, I dream it's a Cheating Day and I'm
romping in a beautiful field of cheeseburgers and whirling Danishes.

As reality creeps in—yes, Goldberg,
it's a *Diet Day*! I'm suddenly being chased
by an angry scale. So what? I'm ready, baby.
I can still chew something good to eat. I can
even have fantasies of delicious diet foods.

Tighten your belt and come along for a
bite-by-bite Goldberg gallup through one
whole Diet Day. Yes, the whole truth of the
way I eat and exercise. Ready? Forward
march to the kitchen faucet.

Gurgling down two twelve-ounce
glasses of cold tap water along with a tablespoon of wheat bran (which is like swallow-

ing a tablespoon of dried, pulverized tree bark), I start my day.

Actually, they're not glasses. They're paper cups. I can throw them out so I don't have to wash 'em. What a lazy slug.

Strolling and looking around my kitchen, I don't think I could get a picture spread in *Better Homes and Gardens*. For some dumb reason, the carriage house (fancy name for horse shed) where I live, did not come with a stove. I don't need a stove. I don't like to cook anyway. I love to make pizzas. So when the pizza madness comes over me, I run to other folks' houses and mess up their kitchens.

Looking at my cooking equipment, the stuff doesn't look like it jumped off the pages of a Williams-Sonoma catalog. I do have a crumb-encrusted GE toaster oven to heat up my bagels and a J.C. Penney microwave oven that has more controls than a Boeing 747. Of course, I only use the timer and the high setting. My kitchen is completed by an electric tea kettle to boil water for my instant coffee.

The door of my warped wooden cabinet creaks when I open it. Inside are two slim, angry moths staring at me. On the shelves are twenty-one foil pizza pans. Eleven mismatched jelly glasses, a skillet for making fortune cookies, a dented stainless-steel bowl for my cereal, and a cheese-dripped rack that I used to make my latest invention: Goldberg's Pizza Cone. Don't ask.

I don't have any real plates. When I'm dining at home, I whip out my elegant designer paper plates.

Eating is much more fun than cooking. Reading cookbooks makes me hungry and bored. Plus cooking takes too long. When I'm hungry, I want to eat *now*! There are plenty of great cooks putting half a teaspoon of cilantro in some twenty-three-ingredient recipe, but not yours truly. I'm just a pizza man, plain and simple.

Probably a breakfast cereal manufacturer once said, you should eat breakfast like a king, lunch like a prince, and dinner like a pauper. Hold on, this is a real sexist saying. What is the queen supposed to eat, a croissant? Anyway, this little sentence has always made sense to me. I love a big breakfast. I'm coming out of a seven-hour sleeping fast and need to stoke the furnace of my hungry body.

Before strapping on the morning feed bag, I like to exercise my sleek body for a little sweaty appetizer.

STATIONARY BIKING

Three or four times a week, I hoist myself on that old standby, my Schwinn Air Dyne stationary bicycle, for thirty fun-filled minutes.

My doctor in New York is a cardiologist and sausage, mushroom, and onion pizza eater who prescribed stand-still biking as one of the best exercises for fitness. So, I took a fistful of bucks and bought my first bike with a speedometer and a dial that increases tension on the wheel. That was about twenty-five years ago.

The Air Dyne is my third stationary bike. I've probably pedaled to the moon and back.

THE NAKED BEDROOM

I plant my one-wheeled torture chamber in the bedroom because it's the one room of my three that has the least action. I do my biking ritual in the nude. Don't get excited. The whole body breathes, keeps cool, and its more fun. If you get a stationary bicycle and want to pedal in the buff, I suggest you get a well-upholstered seat.

THE GOOD NEWS

When I exercise on a bike that goes nowhere, I can exercise any time I feel twitchy, blah, or sluggish. I can move the bike out to the driveway, front yard, or in the living room when I'm entertaining— with my clothes on, of course.

I can forget about thunderstorms, blizzards, cold, heat, snapping dogs, falling meteors, foot and knee problems, space aliens, sunburn, and muggers.

THE BAD NEWS

Stationary biking is *boring*. I'm convinced boredom was invented on the stationary bike. The only way I can do it without getting hives is:

1. Watching television—I climb on my bike sometime between seven and nine in the morning. The morning shows save my life.
2. Reading—I bought a book rack that fits on the handlebars. *People* magazine is perfect reading.
3. Daydreaming—when nothing else

works and the minutes seem like I'm in a dentist's chair, I go into my Stationary Daydream Trance. There are no Super Bowls I haven't won in the last five seconds; no unfriendly countries I haven't infiltrated as a dashing spy; no movie leading ladies I haven't romanced while winning triple Oscars for best actor, best director, and best screenplay; no Broadway musicals I haven't stopped with my brilliant singing and dancing.

MORE GOOD NEWS

When I hear the bell after thirty minutes, I'm so happy I could kiss a python. My body is charged, every cell is doing a dance, I feel terrific, and my heart is off to a good, pounding start.

After the wonderful workout, I gurgle down another big glass of ice water.

Hooray, it's time for breakfast. What do I eat almost every day?

A BIG BEAUTIFUL BAGEL

Sometimes, just as I wake up, I have a vision of a gigantic bagel from heaven, swathed in a blinding halo of cream cheese hovering above my bed.

The bagel is:

- The dieter's pal and my best food friend on Diet Days.
- The unbroken circle of life—no beginning, no end. Take that, Freud.

- Chewy, dense, coarse, filling, and a taste bud dance.
- You can pick from many flavors. Some bagel stores have twenty flavors. I am never bagel bored.
- Low-fat, protein rich, and made with unbleached high gluten flour. What can be better for you?
- Although bagels are best fresh, they can be kept frozen until eating time.
- Bagels take a long time to eat, make strong jaws, and are great for dunking.
- A plain bagel has no cholesterol or artificial coloring.
- Anything can be smeared on it and it tastes great.
- A bagel is a doughnut with brains.
- A bagel is a doughnut dipped in concrete.

So I warm or toast my bagel and squirt a little "I-Can't-Believe-It's-Not-Butter" on it. The bagel loves it. Maybe I add a little jelly or low-fat cream cheese. To round out the meal, I have a big mug of instant Folger's coffee mixed in with Alba Hot Chocolate with Nutrasweet. Gives the coffee a yummy mocha taste. That's my Bagel Breakfast.

BREAKFAST #2:
BIG BOWL OF CEREAL

I choose a whole grain cereal, either cold or hot, like lumpy oatmeal. Eyeballing the ingredients on the package is important. If it includes sugar or salt, I make sure they're low on the list of ingredients. Then I pour on just enough skim milk to cover the cereal yet keep it crunchy.

Grape Nuts are one of my all-time, anytime favorite foods. I know I'm really eating something. When I eat a bowl, the noise of the crunching, popping, and chewing in my head makes it seem like I'm sitting on the stage of a Rolling Stones concert.

Sometimes I mix Grape Nuts with All Bran or Wheaties or I put all three in a washtub.

I love bananas on my cereal. They have to be soft, ripe, with a few brown spots and zipper skins. I like to play with them when they float on top of the milk like little yellow rafts.

BREAKFAST #3: EGGS

I go out for this breakfast about once every three weeks. I have two eggs poached, soft- or hard-boiled, fried, or scrambled. I love my scrambled eggs soft and runny so that I almost need a spoon to get every last morsel.

I can't have eggs without bread. With my eggs, I have one toasted bagel, or one English muffin, or two slices rye or whole wheat toast with margarine. Topped off with diner coffee or tea and a glass of skim milk, this is luxury eating.

I ate basically this same breakfast of ten to fourteen eggs per week for many years because I could look forward to a big breakfast. Man, how I love eggs and a bagel or English muffin.

My egg breakfasts were dynamite until

my doctor discovered that my cholesterol was off the charts, thanks mainly to those golden egg yolks that I soaked up with my bagels.

After I became the Cholesterol King, I seldom eat #3. My cholesterol is now down to 201.

Fruit and vegetable juices never excited me. It's too easy. Give me the whole fruit or vegetable. I like the biting, chewing, and dripping. There's not enough action in drinking, and the filling fiber from the skin is lost.

HOW I EAT THE REST OF MY DIET DAY OR WHO NEEDS LUNCH AND DINNER? NIBBLING, NOSHING, AND GNAWING TO SLIMDOM WITH THE TWO-FINGER EATING PLAN.

I learned two-finger dining watching my pal, Fifi White, a 115-pounder who always eats with two fingers and always says she's fat. *Ha!*

Two-finger eating is nibbling on only as much food you can hold between your thumb and index finger.

Strong fingers don't count. No fair if you can hold a barbecued side of beef between your thumb and forefinger.

Watching slim folks eat can earn your master's degree in losing weight and keeping it off. Fatty see, fatty do.

I've chewed on wooden toothpicks and Stim-U-Dents for years. They're great adult pacifiers when I'm hungry. I think my teeth have termites.

I hate feeling hungry, so I eat little bites all day long.

Nibbling is fun and I get lots more, different flavors exploding behind my teeth.

Who said you had to have three "square" meals a day?

I get bored eating the same food all the time.

BOREDOM IS THE DEATH OF DIETING!

I LOVE SANDWICHES . . .

Especially turkey, lean roast beef, or water-packed tuna. Tuna fish is great mixed with a teaspoon of low-fat Miracle Whip, celery, onions, and a teaspoon of sweet pickle relish. I like to pile the stuff on rye, whole grain, or pumpernickel bread or bagels.

Smear on the mustard or a teaspoon of Russian dressing with two fingers of cole slaw. No ketchup—too much sugar.

Watch out. The turkey could be turkey roll, which is loaded with salt. I ask for fresh, roasted turkey. They giggle. After they stop laughing, I ask for turkey breast. I always demand a taste to check it out.

Sandwiches are great traveling companions.

SALAD BARS

Most salad bars don't make my heart go pitter patter. Remember, Eve picked an apple in the Garden of Eden, not a head of iceberg lettuce. God knew that veggies were no temptation.

If you crave a salad, supermarkets and fast-food cafés have good salad bars. I must confess I think salads are for sissies. But I'm getting better. When I'm really hungry, even salads taste good. Call me half a sissy!

BAKED POTATO BARS

Baked potatoes are a diet life saver. I eat them all over the city or I nuke 'em in my microwave. I eat them straight or with a squirt of olive oil or margarine, a bit of low-fat cottage cheese or plain yogurt with chives, or a dusting of Parmesan cheese, or anything else that's low fat.

I like the skins, too. It takes a while to get used to microwaved skins, but keep on chewing.

Potatoes look like a Big Bertha Bomb. That's what they feel like when they drop in my tummy. But I'm full and happy for a long time.

I eat with my eyes, too. Maybe my eyes are gaining weight.

About six or seven in the evening is as late as I like to eat on a Diet Day.

POPCORN

Pop, pop, pop, popular, perfect popcorn: tasty, noisy, takes a long time to eat with two fingers, low-fat, low-calorie, cheap, fiber-rich, nutritious, and chewy. I bought one of those hot air popcorn poppers when I found out that popcorn, when it's not popped in oils, is extra low cal.

I quick-walk a half hour a day.

I don't count calories. Counting those things is overrated, inaccurate, and numbers drive me crazy. I eat by portion and fat content.

Water is my queen every day. I drink eight to ten glasses. Those plastic bottles with the hose in the top help me slurp while schlepping.

Bread is the staff of my life. Whoever heard about a food riot over a shortage of brussels sprouts?

On Diet Days, I try to eat fresh, natural, and simple.

Cafe Lulu in Kansas City, where I work, has delicious, healthy food, and is an oasis of fun. Yes, this is a plug.

Houston's Restaurant (I don't work there) has a grilled chicken salad that will knock your socks off. Get the dressing on the side. This huge baby takes forty-five minutes of hard-driving chewing. I actually lose weight in my jaw, and I'm going to join the circus as one of the guys who can hang by their teeth and spin around.

HAPPY HOURS

Smart, enterprising restaurateurs, for a dollar or two, give the after-work crowd a large table groaning with mountains of eats.

This lavish spread is supposed to keep the gang drinking Pepsi, hanging out, mingling, and gnawing on chicken wings and carrot sticks. Usually there's a large vegetable medley that has no takers. This is where I eat a lot of my veggies. I buy a $2.50 bottle of fancy faucet water from France, grab a handful of cauliflower, and look for a wife.

Hey, fellow vegetable haters, I found a great way for us to eat our greens . . . I'm so nervous chatting with a good-looking woman, I don't know that I'm eating iceberg lettuce.

ROLLING MY OWN AT HOME

I'm a great food assembler, bringer-inner, defroster, heater-upper, and jar opener. The microwave oven was invented for me. The only thing it can't do with food is buy it. Corn on the cob is my favorite. Especially when it's homegrown. The sweet corn kernels stick between my teeth. I can play with those for hours.

The supermarket freezer is turning into a health food store. Lots of low-fat, low-sodium, frozen meals that are truly tasty. And you can pick from so many varieties. Since my Indian name is "He Who Never Cooks," diet dining has never been this easy.

What's sweet, juicy, sloppy, slurpy, nutritious, almost no calories, and takes a long time to eat? Melons, of course. I'm a melon head. Any melon is my meat. One question. How do I get cantaloupes from smelling up my ice box? I love all kinds of fruits, especially bananas. Maybe I'm a fruitarian.

MY REFRIGERATOR

THE FREEZER

My freezer is a library of some of the greatest bagels ever produced. It is stuffed with Pumpernickel raisin bagels from Ess-A-Bagel in New York's Lower East Side; "Black Russians," a coarse black bagel with fresh onions topped with sesame seeds, from Jumbo Bagel in NYC; Cinnamon Raisin bagels from Bagel & Bagel in Kansas City.

For my Cheating Day, nestled between the bagels, is a glazed "twist" from Lamar's Donuts in Kansas City. Without a doubt, the best bakery in the world.

A twist is a deep-fried extravaganza the size of a small baseball bat. This is my "Field of Dreams." It is a foot long, weighs half a pound, and covers the three food groups on Cheating Days: grease, dough, and sugar. Come to KC and I'll introduce you to Raymond Lamar.

TOP SHELF

- ¼ squeeze bottle of I-Can't-Believe-It's-Not-Butter
- ¾ jar of Smucker's Grape Jelly
- A Rubbermaid container of wheat bran

MIDDLE SHELF

- Three bottles of barbecue sauce: Arthur Bryant's, K.C. Masterpiece, and Marty's
- ½ gallon skim milk
- Two squeeze bottles of mustard
- Five homegrown Jonathan apples
- Two red Bartlett pears
- One shriveled pink grapefruit

BOTTOM SHELF, VEGETABLE CRISPER, DOOR SHELVES

* empty

ON TOP OF THE REFRIGERATOR

* seven bananas of various stages of ripeness

Sometimes it pays to be a single guy on a diet. I only have to defrost and clean the refrigerator once a year.

THE RAIDER OF THE LOST REFRIGERATOR
OR
EATING IN OTHER FOLKS' REFRIGERATORS
(The best place to eat on a Diet Day)

STARRING
Hungry Berg as Missouri Jones

When a pal or a stranger opens the door of his house, I run straight to the ice box.

OFR (Other Folks' Refrigerators) always have loads of foil- and plastic-wrapped untold food riches waiting for my hungry hands.

Rummaging through the cold shelves is like finding Christmas or Chanukah presents. I don't forget the back of the fridge either. You never know where they hide the good stuff.

If I'm lucky, there's a foil-wrapped, leftover prime rib or roast chicken, or a whole, slightly used turkey carcass, with meat all over that the carving knife couldn't get.

One good turkey leg, a bottle of Durkee's dressing, and eating over the sink, is heaven.

I don't miss those containers with lids, either. I always open them up. Could be tuna fish, rice and beans, or melon balls.

I don't look in the freezer. It takes too long to thaw out frozen food. That would be rude.

I could live the rest of my life on leftovers.

Oh boy. There is one danger to refrigerator grazing. Eating someone's lunch can be tricky.

CAR CUISINE

The automobile and I have had an eating love affair for all my born days. There have been seven beautiful cars in my past, and now that I'm back in KC I'm on the streets again with a 1986 roadster.

My favorite dining room is inside my car. Thanks to drive-thrus, food trays, soda pop containers, flat seats, and cheap paper towels, I can eat anything while driving, including watermelon. During watermelon season, the seeds get so deep on the floor, I sweep out my car at least twice a week.

I am confident that I can eat in any restaurant or beanery and get something good and healthy. My motto on Diet Days is, "DON'T ACT DUMB, GOLDBERG." Don't con yourself, don't try to make deals. You know what to eat and NOT EAT.

"Hello there, Big Boy. Why don't you

come join me for a little while?" purr the Grease, Dough, and Sugar Sirens. I totally ignore those temptresses on Diet Days. Take that, you hussies.

If I'm not hungry, I DON'T EAT.

I eat breakfast anytime.

I seldom eat red meat on Diet Days.

AEROBIC DANCING

I love to impersonate Gene Kelly and Fred Astaire. So, several times a week I do aerobic dancing at Susie Brown's Body Trends in KC. My heart pounds not only from the workout but from watching beautiful women jumping up and down in tight Spandex costumes.

DINING ON THE SIDEWALKS, STREETS, AND SUBWAYS

With twenty-one years practice in New York City, I can eat whole meals walking fast, talking loud, and not getting run over by a cab. That's why I love hand foods, delis, and pizza slices.

GOLDBERG'S RULES:

- If you eat sitting down, you gain weight.
- If you eat standing up, you're even.
- If you eat while walking, you lose weight.

INGREDIENT AND NUTRITION LABELING OR SHOPPING WITH FATS

Here we go to the grocery store. Grab one of those 450-pound carts that has a bad wheel and goes sideways. Before we put anything in the cart:

1. Read all food labels as though they were the front page of the *National Enquirer*, INTENSELY.
2. Look for the serving size and how many servings are in the package.
3. Check out the nutritional labeling for calories and fats. Also see how nutritious the product is for your money. Don't waste your money on high-priced phooey foods.
4. Remember, on the ingredient label, the ingredients are listed from most to least.
5. I line up similar products on a vacant shelf looking for the least fat content, sugar, sodium, and calories. Sometimes, I see the manager watching me from behind the Clorox.
6. Don't go to the grocery store if you're hungry or in a hurry.
7. Plan what you're going to eat. Make a list. No impulse buying, you money bags, you.
8. You're single? Hang out in the produce department. The word is this place could be a hot spot to find a sweetie pie.

As I'm writing this on a sunny, Sunday afternoon, November 11, 1990, the Feds just passed a new food-labeling law that eliminates gimmicks and confusion. But it will be a while before the new food labeling is enacted.

Right now, you are governed by the
Goldberg food-labeling law:
CHECK EVERY LABEL.

READING THOSE LABELS

INGREDIENT LABELS

Adjust the bifocals and read the fine
print on the labels when you buy stuff at the
grocery. Labels can help you make smart
food choices. We all know that you're a
smarty pants. Even better, compare labels
of the same goods so you can choose foods
that are lowest in fats, cholesterol, calories,
sugar, and salt.

On the label, the ingredients are listed
by their weight, from most to least. The
label won't give you the exact amount of
any ingredient, but you can figure it out. If
fat, sugar, or salt (sodium) is listed first or
second, then you can bet your bottom Oreo
that the food is loaded with that particular
ingredient.

FATS

Check out the following list of saturated fat and cholesterol sources, so you can
spot them on labels: animal fat, lard, coconut oil, coconut palm oil, palm oil, palm
kernel oil, whole milk solids, cocoa butter,
egg and egg yolk solids, butter, cream, and
hydrogenated vegetable oil.

Cholesterol is a fatlike substance that
clogs your arteries. It's found in foods of
animal origin, such as egg yolks, meat,
poultry, fish, and dairy products. Foods of
plant origin, such as fruits, vegetables,

grains, nuts, seeds, dry beans and peas, and vegetable oils have no cholesterol.

SUGARS

Surprise, there are many more sugars than the white granulated sucrose sugar sitting in grandma's sugar bowl on the kitchen table. Watch out for these on those labels: glucose, dextrose, fructose, maltose, lactose, sorbitol, mannitol, honey, corn syrup, molasses, and maple syrup.

SALT AND SODIUM

Look for any listed ingredient that has "salt" or "sodium" in the name.

NUTRITIONAL LABELING

The feds require nutritional labeling on food products that have added nutrients or nutritional claims. The poop on the nutritional labeling is divided into two categories:

1. "Nutrition Information per Serving" Serving size, number of servings per container, calories per serving, protein, carbohydrates, fat, and sodium per serving in grams.
2. "Percentage of the U.S. Recommended Daily Allowance" This will show the percentage of protein, five vitamins, and two minerals provided in a serving.

Be careful when you compare nutritional labels. The manufacturer chooses the

serving size. These can vary from product
to product.

THE FDA DICTIONARY

Okay, dear dieter, when you see the
following words on a label, it's important to
know what they mean. These are the defini-
tions according to the U.S. Food and Drug
Administration regulations:

> *Cholesterol Free:* Less than 2 milli-
> grams of cholesterol per serving.
> *Low Cholesterol:* Less than 20 milli-
> grams per serving.
> *Reduced Cholesterol:* 75 percent less
> cholesterol than is normally found
> in the food.
> *Sodium Free:* Less than 5 milligrams of
> sodium per serving.
> *Very Low Sodium:* 35 milligrams or less
> per serving.
> *Low Sodium:* 140 milligrams or less
> per serving.
> *Unsalted, Without Added Salt, or No
> Salt Added:* Made without the salt
> that's normally used.
> *Low-Calorie:* Contains no more than
> 40 calories per serving.
> *Reduced Calorie:* At least one-third
> fewer calories than the regular prod-
> uct. (For example, reduced-calorie
> salad dressing in place of regular
> salad dressing.)

Also, don't assume "diet" and "dietetic" mean low in calories. These terms
mean a food has been changed in some way.

The change might be fewer calories, less sodium, less cholesterol, or a different type of sugar than in the regular product. Read that label to find out exactly what the "diet" claim means.

SEEING THE LIGHT ON LITE

Except for meat and poultry, no regulations now exist that define light and "lite." Manufacturers have interpreted these terms to mean anything from lower in calories, fat, or sodium, to lighter in color or flavor. The weird part is that "Lite" products sometimes cost more than regular products. So, before you stock up, make sure you compare calories, fat, sodium, and cost of these foods with their regular counterparts.

THE LAST WORD: THE SLIM EVANGELIST SPEAKS

FROM THE TEMPLE
OF CONTROLLED CHEATING
AND HEAVENLY THINNESS
SERMON: 11:00 A.M.
"HELP FOR THE HEAVY"

You are fat! Yesiree, brothers and sisters, sisters and brothers, you are obese!

There you sit in the ice box, eating yourselves into oblivion. You're never going up to heaven. Do you know why? Because no one can lift you, that's why.

Are you tired of being called a nice couple? Are you wearing your old necklace as a wedding ring? Can you be saved? Yes, yes, and amen.

Who will help you lay down that knife and fork and walk that slim path? I will, Brother Fats.

Now turn to page forty-three in your Sara Lee hymnal, and we will sing "Shut My Mouth."

"We're gonna leave our bags of candy bars . . .
down by the riverside . . .

down by the riverside.
We're gonna leave our cakes and cookie
jars . . .
down by the riverside . . .
ain't gonna stuff our mouths no more."

(And when we finish our hymns, we say
"Amen," not "Pass the Plate.")
Sisters and brothers, I've been fat and
I've been skinny. And I'm here to tell you
skinny is better. Do I hear a HALLELUJAH!
I haven't forgotten what it's like in the
land of dunking doughnuts and peanut brittle.
I haven't forgotten those wild times at
the five-stool joints with the great greasy
bacon cheeseburgers, pancake houses where
warm maple syrup and butter flow out of
faucets, and Mexican palaces where the com-
bination platters have enough combined calo-
ries to give a computer a hernia.
No, no, no. I haven't forgotten any of
that big-time eating. How can I forget? I've
gone all through the fiery hells of fatness just
like you have, sisters and brothers.
Say it with me, now. No more fatness.
Louder. NO MORE FATNESS! Can I
have a gigantic AMEN for NO MORE
FATNESS!
I've crawled on my belly, hands, and
knees, begging to be taken out in a snowstorm
for a dozen hot sticky glazed doughnuts and a
quart of cold chocolate milk.
I've screamed up to heaven for a torren-
tial downpour of walnut brownies and vanilla
ice cream. Then one day, lying in the gutter
filled with pepperoni pizza, I cried for some-
one to help me lose weight and keep it off.

Miracle of miracles, a big strong hand took my shoulder and helped me to my shaky feet. A thundering voice came from I-know-not-where, booming, "You and you alone, Goldberg, are responsible for the way you eat."

Looking around in a heavenly daze, I discovered that the helping hand and voice came from me, *from deep inside* my *soul. I deliberated, I meditated, and then it happened.*

From the supermarket in my mind came the biggest, best food package of all—Controlled Cheating. The answer from heaven for the desperate dieter. A chock-full-of-wisdom way to lose weight. Now and forever.

THE FIVE COMMANDMENTS OF CONTROLLED CHEATING

Controlled Cheating is THE answer to losing weight and keeping it off. Dear brothers and sisters, you may rightly ask, how?

1. I know Controlled Cheating works because I am sitting and writing this on a cold morning in November. A fat guy who wasn't supposed to be around past the age of thirty, here I am cavorting and playing in my Nike shoes, a happy fifty-seven-year-old, and in perfect health (except for one corn, two varicose veins, and one pair of bifocal glasses).

   Controlled Cheating works. I lost 175 pounds and have kept it off for thirty-two years. When all else failed in my fat-eating life, Cheating Eating rescued me from the hellish depths of hot butterscotch sauce.

2. Controlled Cheating works because it is a program, plan, road map, and system. Look at every success you've had, in spite of the odds. It had a system. Everything must have a system, a clear individual program that you follow, working or playing. With a good plan, everything you desire and want to accomplish will be possible to achieve.

3. Controlled Cheating works because you have complete control over everything you eat, including the days you are going to cheat and eat. This completely eliminates guilt and depression. The tremendous burden of always having to think about what and where you're going to cheat has disappeared.

Hold on. Hold on. Do I see a repenting brother stumbling off the sawdust trail of Controlled Cheating? Say it, brother. Say what's in your heart. Confess your calories.

"I'm hooked on chocolate, Brother Fats. I can't help myself. My folks never loved me. The first kiss they gave me was a Hershey. From then on, I knew where to find love. But soon plain chocolate wasn't enough. I wanted chocolate-covered raisins, candy bars with almonds! Malteds! Pies! Anything! I can't hold a job. I weigh three hundred pounds. My skin's broken out. And to top it all off, my wife ran away. Oh, help me, somebody's got to help me, Brother Fats. What'll I do? What'll I do?"

It's very simple. Stop eating chocolate every day of the week—but one.

(Amazed.) "Gee, I never thought of that. Thank you, brother. Bless you. Just stop eating chocolate six days a week. You're an amazing man, Brother Fats. Stop eating chocolate until the seventh day and then, *bam*! Boy, he's everything they said he was."

Thank you, brother. Chocolate lives!

4. Controlled Cheating works because it makes you laugh and have fun. On your Cheating Eating Days every week, you can play and have good things to eat. Plus you learn that **Bozo, Crazy, Uncontrolled Cheating Does Not Work.**

5. Controlled Cheating works because everyone and their basset hound is going to cheat. Cheating is as natural as the sunrise and is the concrete foundation of the Controlled Cheating program.

Controlled Cheating is part of our humanness. We all need and deserve a day of rest from hard work, especially the brutally hard work of losing weight and keeping it off.

I quote now from The Holy Scriptures, according to the Masoretic Text from The Jewish Publication Society of America, the Book of Genesis, 2:1-3:

"And the heaven and earth were finished, and all the host of them. And on the seventh day God finished His work which He had made; and He rested on the seventh day from all His work which He had made. And God blessed the seventh day, and hallowed it; because that in it He rested from all His work which God in creating had made."

Good luck and keep eating!

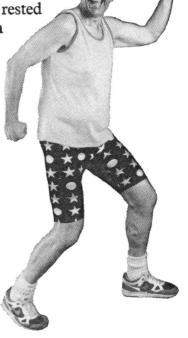